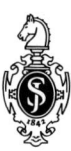

Eugen Plas (ed.)

Heinz Pflüger, Ulrich Maier,
Wilhelm Hübner (co. eds.)

The Aging Bladder

SpringerWienNewYork

Eugen Plas, M.D., F.E.B.U.
Associate Professor of Urology, Department of Urology, Lainz Hospital and LBI for Urology and Andrology, Vienna, Austria

Heinz Pflüger, M.D.
Professor of Urology, Department of Urology, Lainz Hospital and LBI for Urology and Andrology, Vienna, Austria

Ulrich Maier, M.D.†
Professor of Urology, Department of Urology and Andrology, Donauspital, Vienna, Austria

Wilhelm A. Hübner, M.D.
Associate Professor of Urology, Department of Urology, Humanis Klinikum Korneuburg, Korneuburg, Austria

© 2004 Springer-Verlag/Wien
Printed in Austria

Typesetting: Thomson Press (India) Ltd., Chennai, India
Printing: Grasl Druck & Neue Medien, A-2540 Bad Vöslau

Printed on acid-free and chlorine-free bleached paper
SPIN: 10882187

With 61 partly coloured Figures

CIP data applied for

ISBN 3-211-83858-9 Springer-Verlag Wien New York

To Ulrich Maier,

who has been a friend and teacher. He will remain in our minds as an empathetic clinician with constant interest in new perspectives and developments in urology.

Preface

Aging – we are confronted with aging everyday, either personally or in our daily clinical practice. Although aging is a normal process in nature, we become aware of age once we experience changes of body shape, fitness, activity, physical infirmities or diseases. Although everyone experiences aging, each individual is differently affected by the aging process. The way in which mental or physical infirmities affect someone is closely related to that individual's expectancies of life, i.e. expectations that each individual attaches to certain periods of life. As long as changes are in a balanced interaction with personal expectations, people are usually not affected by them. Once people start to experience an imbalance of expectations and personal feelings they become affected by these changes.

Over the past 200 years tremendous technical and medical developments and improvements in daily life have enabled mankind to extend life expectancy notably. The increase in life expectancy is a worldwide trend that is closely associated with an increase in comorbidity of various diseases such as coronary heart disease, metabolic and endocrine disorders, osteoporosis, cancer, and diseases of the genitourinary tract. Although much progress has been made in the past century to improve the health of the aging population, numerous unresolved questions still remain.

One major aspect associated with aging is the development of symptoms of the lower genitourinary tract. Increasing irritative and obstructive voiding symptoms both for men and for women occur with age and are often combined with urinary tract infections. Although these changes usually do not terminate life, they can have an appreciable impact on the quality of life for the aging men and women. They affect daily life – shopping, for example, has to be planned in minute detail according to the availability of toilets; visits to cultural events can be undertaken only with hesitation, and even travelling can be limited owing to fear of incontinence. These changes affect quality of life negatively, especially in a society that is health and body fitness oriented. In addition to personal aspects, changes of bladder function in aging people may require some form of medication or incontinence devices that place a high burden on healthcare budgets.

Successful treatment will clearly have a significant impact on the quality of life for elderly people. It was the aim of this comprehensive book to review current knowledge on anatomical, functional, diagnostic, and therapeutic aspects of the aging bladder associated with closely related issues such as bowel function in elderly people and endocrine changes of the hypophysis, testis, and ovaries with their possible influence on bladder function. Besides state of the art presentations of the aging bladder I am hoping to increase doctors' awareness and interest on the important topic of the aging bladder to advance scientific efforts worldwide on different aspects of the aging bladder.

Much work has already been done, and I am very glad about and grateful for the participation of well known experts in their fields and their preparation of comprehensive manuscripts. As I have learned from many discussions during this project, the combination of different aspects and knowledge of experts opens one's mind, creating new ideas and thoughts for improving the treatment of our patients. I hope that readers will gain an overview and find interesting new aspects that may initiate progress in the treatment of the aging bladder.

I am also very grateful to my mentors Professor Heinz Pflüger, MD and Associate Professor Wilhelm A. Hübner, MD for intense and continuous discussions and for their support during the past ten years, all of which have made urology for me such a broad and open field. Not only did I gain a lot of knowledge, I was trained not to forget the principles of Hippocrates even in a time of continuous medical progress: "It is the patient to be treated, not the disease."

Additionally, I would like to thank Sylvia Seefried, MA for her support during preparation of this book and my wife Katharina for supporting my enthusiasm for and enjoyment of my profession.

Vienna, July 2003

Eugen Plas, MD

Contents

Contributors

Karl-Erik Andersson, MD, PhD, Professor and Chairman, Department of Clinical Pharmacology, Institute for Laboratory Medicine, Lund University Hospital, S-221 85 Lund, Sweden

Sami Arap, MD, Professor and Chairman, Division of Urology, University of São Paulo School of Medicine, Rua Barata Ribeiro, 237 cjs. 104–106, 01308-000 São Paulo-SP, Brazil

Lukas K. Daha, MD, Department of Urology and LBI for Urology & Andrology, Lainz Hospital Vienna, Wolkersbergenstrasse 1, A-1130 Vienna, Austria

Jens-Christian Djurhuus, MD, DMSc, Professor and Chairman, International Enuresis Research Center, Institute of Experimental Clinical Research, Skejby Hospital, Brendstrupgardsvej, DK-8200 Aarhus N, Denmark

Paul C. Dolber, PhD, Co-Director, NeuroUrology Research, Box 3453, Duke University Medical Center, Durham, NC 27710, USA

Johann Hammer, MD, Associate Professor, Department of Gastroenterology and Hepatology, University Clinic of Internal Medicine IV, General Hospital of Vienna, Währinger Gürtel 18–20, A-1090 Vienna, Austria

Christian Hampel, MD, Assistant Professor, Department of Urology, Johannes Gutenberg University Mainz, Langenbeckstrasse 1, D-55131 Mainz, Germany

Christof van der Horst, MD, Department of Urology, University of Schleswig-Holstein – Campus Kiel, Arnold-Heller-Strasse 7, D-24105 Kiel, Germany

Wilhelm A. Hübner, MD, Associate Professor and Chairman, Department of Urology, Klinikum Weinviertel, Wiener Ring 3-4, A-2100 Korneuburg, Austria

Gitte M. Hvistendahl, MD, Senior registrar, International Enuresis Research Center, Institute of Experimental Clinical Research, Skejby Hospital, Brendstrupgardsvej, DK-8200 Aarhus N, Denmark

Klaus P. Jünemann, MD, Professor and Chairman, Department of Urology, University of Schleswig-Holstein – Campus Kiel, Arnold-Heller-Strasse 7, D-24105 Kiel, Germany

Cynthia M. Kuhn, PhD, Professor of Pharmacology, 401-I Bryan Research Building, Department of Surgery, Duke University Medical Center, Durham, NC 27710, USA

Ulrich Maier, MD[†], Professor and Chairman, Department of Urology and Andrology, Sozialmedizinisches Zentrum Ost – Donauspital, Langobardenstrasse 122, A-1220 Vienna, Austria

Cristiano Mendes Gomes, MD, Assistant Professor, Division of Urology, University of São Paulo School of Medicine, Rua Barata Ribeiro, 237 cjs. 104–106, 01308-000 São Paulo-SP, Brazil

Heinz Pflüger, MD, Professor and Chairman, Department of Urology and LBI for Urology & Andrology, Lainz Hospital Vienna, Wolkersbergenstrasse 1, A-1130 Vienna Austria

Eugen Plas, MD, Associate Professor, Department of Urology and LBI for Urology & Andrology, Lainz Hospital Vienna, Wolkersbergenstrasse 1, A-1130 Vienna, Austria

Claus Riedl, MD, Associate Professor and Chairman, Department of Urology, Thermenklinikum Baden, Wimmergasse 19, A-2500 Baden, Austria

Dorothea Rohrmann, MD, Associate Professor, Department of Urology, Universitätsklinikum Aachen, Pauwelsstrasse 30, D-52057 Aachen, Germany

Manfred Schmidbauer, MD, Professor and Chairman, Department of Neurology, Lainz Hospital, Wolkersbergenstrasse 1, A-1130 Vienna, Austria

Debra A. Schwinn, MD, Professor of Anesthesiology, Professor of Surgery, Professor of Pharmacology/Cancer Biology, Vice Chairman for Research, 105 Sands Building, Duke University Medical Center, Durham, NC 27710, USA

Martin Susani, MD, Professor, Department of Clinical Pathology, University of Vienna, General Hospital of Vienna, Währinger Gürtel 18–20, A-1090 Vienna, Austria

Karl B. Thor, PhD, Co-Director, NeuroUrology Research, Box 3453, Duke University Medical Center, Durham, NC 27710, USA

Joachim W. Thüroff, MD, Professor and Chairman, Department of Urology, Johannes Gutenberg University Mainz, Langenbeckstrasse 1, D-55131 Mainz, Germany

Flavio Trigo-Rocha, MD, Associate Professor, Head-Section of Urodynamics, Division of Urology, University of São Paulo School of Medicine, Rua Barata Ribeiro, 237 cjs. 104–106, 01308-000 São Paulo-SP, Brazil

Anatomy and pathophysiology of the aging bladder

C. van der Horst and *K.-P. Jünemann*

Department of Urology, University of Schleswig-Holstein –
Campus Kiel, Kiel, Germany

Contents

1.   Introduction

Bladder function and dysfunction in elderly people differ from those in younger adults. Impairment of bladder function, such as detrusor instability or urinary retention, may occur alone or in combination with urinary incontinence. To identify the cause of each dysfunctional pattern, both the morphological and the physiological changes in the aging bladder need to be investigated, in particular the changes in the function of the lower urinary tract and its central control. Voiding disorders in elderly people are rarely related to isolated specific anatomical or physiological changes; most commonly, they are the result of several interacting factors which may include medication (particularly centrally acting agents), immobility, metabolic imbalances, and previous surgical procedures, as well as cerebrospinal degeneration and disease (Jünemann 2000).

Elderly patients often have an uncontrolled micturition reflex. At full bladder capacity, an abrupt sensation occurs and cannot be controlled appropriately. If the toilet cannot be reached within a few minutes the patient becomes incontinent. Although the urodynamic pattern of such patients corresponds with the pattern shown by an uninhibited neuropathic bladder dysfunction (involuntary detrusor contraction), the original patho-physiology of the so-called idiopathic detrusor overactivity is still unknown (Melchior 1995).

Only few, but none the less specific, anatomical differences exist between the female and the male bladder. In men the prostate gland, as a potentially obstructive organ, and in women the pelvic floor, which may become insufficiently strong after childbirth or through fluctuation of oestrogen, may rise to specific problems. Prostate hypertrophy or malignancy may cause bladder outflow obstruction with lower urinary tract symptoms (LUTS) and can result in urge- or overflow-incontinence. After surgery for prostate cancer, stress incontinence is the predominant mode of dysfunction in most patients (Moore 1999).

Stress incontinence in women has been investigated by multiple groups, but an understanding of its pathophysiology was provided by the work of Petros and Ulmsten (1990). In their "integration theory", an anatomical defect reported as "slack vagina" was identified as the major reason for stress incontinence in women. According to their hypothesis, this slackness may be caused by defects in the vaginal wall itself and its supporting structures, such as ligaments, muscles, and connective tissue insertions. Additionally, Petros and Ulmsten described an alteration of collagen and elastin in the vaginal connective tissue and its ligamentous supports, which may be related to the process of aging. Snooks et al. (1984) reported terminal motor latencies to the urethral striated sphincter musculature in patients with faecal and stress incontinence. They provided evidence of damage to the innervation of the urethral striated sphincter musculature in double incontinence. Their results indicate that stress incontinence associated with idiopathic faecal incontinence is due to damage to the nerve supply of the urethral striated sphincter, particularly of the periurethral striated sphincter musculature but also of the intramural striated musculature. They postulated that the somatic efferent innervation of the urethral striated sphincter musculature may also be damaged in patients with isolated stress incontinence. Furthermore, investigations on terminal latency of the pudendal nerve in 50 women 48–72 hours post partum and 8 weeks after delivery, combined with single fibre electromyography (EMG) of the external anal sphincter were performed (Snooks et al. 1984). An increased terminal motor latency of the pudendal nerve was seen in 42% of women 48–72 hours after vaginal delivery but not in women after caesarean section. Damage to the pudendal nerve was more common and severe in multiparous women after vaginal delivery. Single-fibre electromyography of the pelvic floor muscles in later studies found a significantly higher degree of denervation of the pelvic floor in women with urinary stress incontinence, genitourinary prolapse, or both, than in asymptomatic women (Smith et al. 1989a, b). These results indicate that partial denervation of the pelvic floor with subsequent re-innervation (wallerian degeneration) is a common finding after vaginal delivery, which increases with aging.

Additionally, sex hormones have substantial influence on women's lower urinary tract throughout life, with fluctuations in serum concentrations resulting in anatomical, histological, and functional changes (Hextall et al. 2001a). Oestrogen deficiency – as a result of menopause – is associated with a wide range of urogenital complaints, including urge syndrome, nocturia, incontinence, and urinary tract infection (Hextall et al. 2001b, Jackson et al. 1996, Schreiter et al. 1976). Although alterations due to local oestrogen deficiency have been investigated, the influence of oestrogen on the cerebral control of the lower urinary tract is still unclear.

In both sexes, external and internal influences on the anatomy, neuroanatomy, and physiology of the lower urinary tract vary in the aging process.

2.   Anatomy

2.1   The bladder neck

Morphological fundamentals and functional anatomy of urinary continence of the lower urinary tract are still a matter of controversy (Jünemann 2001a). The "musculus sphincter urethrae" is the equivalent of the internal sphincter or sphincter of the bladder neck; the "musculus sphincter vesicae" is the equivalent of the external sphincter or "rhabdosphincter urethrae". These have both been described and accepted in different histopathological studies (Dorschner et al. 2001, Elbadawi et al. 1997b, Myers et al. 1987, Strasser et al. 1996). According to Dorschner et al. (2001) investigating 50 male and 15 female autopsy specimens (all ages including newborn and elderly), the musculus sphincter urethrae or internal sphincter is a circular, distinct structure, which elliptically embraces the internal urethral orifice, and the lamellas of the detrusor are not involved in the formation of the internal sphincter. Controversial to these results are studies from Hinman concerning anatomy of the bladder neck, especially in elderly people (Hinman 1993) which are in context with ours. Figure 1 a shows sagittal histology of the bladder neck region. There are few circular muscle fibres ventral to the prostate, in contrast to the large number of circular muscle fibres at the cranio-dorsal aspect of the prostate, and dorsal to the urethra. The muscular bladder neck region is consistent with the clinical situation of a tight bladder neck, constantly associated with a fixed dorsal part of the bladder neck, and resulting in urinary outflow obstruction. It is remarkable that the histology of the muscles in the area of the bladder neck does not differ with respect to young and old patients. The bladder neck becomes stiff and hypercontractile, without evidence of hypertrophic muscle cells. The only age-related change in the bladder neck is an increasing share of prostatic adenoma cells in the musculus sphincter urethae during aging (Dorschner et al. 2001). This may result from prostatic hyperplasia and is probably not related to the clinical situation of a stiff bladder neck. There are also longitudinal fibres originating from the trigone area, stretching to the colliculus seminalis, according to the base plate theory (Hutch 1967, Tanagho et al. 1966). Nevertheless, the functional anatomy of this region

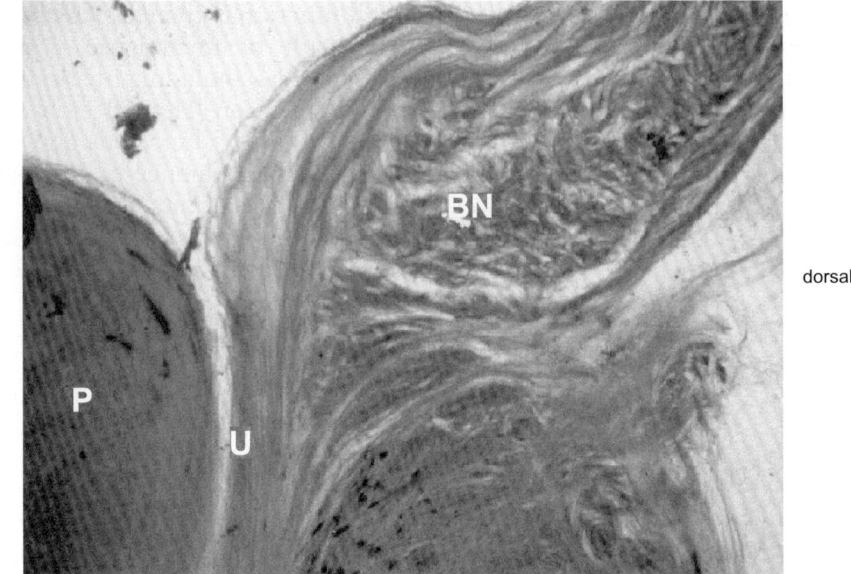

Fig. 1. *P* Prostate; *U* Urethra with longitudinal muscle structure; *BN* Bladder neck with circular muscular structure. There is no muscular structure on the upper surface of the prostate. Dorsal to the urethra is a mass of circular orientated muscles. The longitudinal orientated muscular structures arise from the trigonum vesicae and pass through the prostate into the colliculus (reprinted with permission, Jünemann et al. 2001a)

remains unclear leading to speculation of the functional anatomy of the internal musculus sphincter urethrae.

The neurophysiological results of Dixon and Gosling (Dixon and Gosling 1987) address functional aspects of the musculus sphincter urethrae. It was shown that the musculus sphincter urethrae has a different function than previously assumed only on behalf of histomorphological findings. According to their results, electrical stimulation of sympathetic and parasympathetic nerve fibres led to different responses of the bladder neck and prostate. Their theory of a non-continence related, strictly sexual function of the bladder neck was supported by Maggi in 1993 suggesting only a prevention of retrograde ejaculation in men (Maggi 1993). However, Dixon and Gosling found no corresponding anatomical structure in women, although these patients commonly suffer from of stress incontinence (Dixon and Gosling 1987). But others suggested that the internal musculus sphincter urethrae contains both sexual and continence function.

Neither the reason for a tight bladder neck leading to an outflow obstruction, nor the mechanisms in preserving continence or causing incontinence are completely understood. In view of the histopathological and neurophysiological findings, it can be speculated that stiffness of the bladder neck may be due to a dysfunction of the lower urinary tract caused by changes in the innervation or neural control in elderly people, but so far no studies have supported this theory.

2.2   Ultrastructural analysis of the detrusor muscle

The light microscopic anatomy of the detrusor smooth muscle does not contain gender differences and has only minor alterations between young and elderly bladder detrusor. It consists of three smooth muscle cell layers.

Pivotal work on ultrastructural changes of the baldder detrusor were performed by Eldbadawi et al. (1997, 1998) on detrusor muscle biopsies taken from healthy, asymptomatic young and old men. No significant differences were seen in young detrusor as compared to elderly man. Further biopsies were taken from men complaining of voiding symptoms or lower urinary tract dysfunctions of varying degrees, such as impaired contractility. Within detrusors with impaired contractility, neuroeffector transmission was impeded or suspended by degenerating axons. Ultrastructurally this was identified by degeneration of smooth muscle cells (Fig. 2) by dissolving intracellular contacts, degeneration and finally apoptosis. As a result, cell detritus was found between degenerated smooth muscle cells.

The histological pattern of a detrusor muscle biopsy in a patient with subvesical outflow obstruction is shown in Fig. 3. The muscular structure is left intact, but the fascicular orientation of the connective tissue is disordered with an increase in connective tissue that compromises the

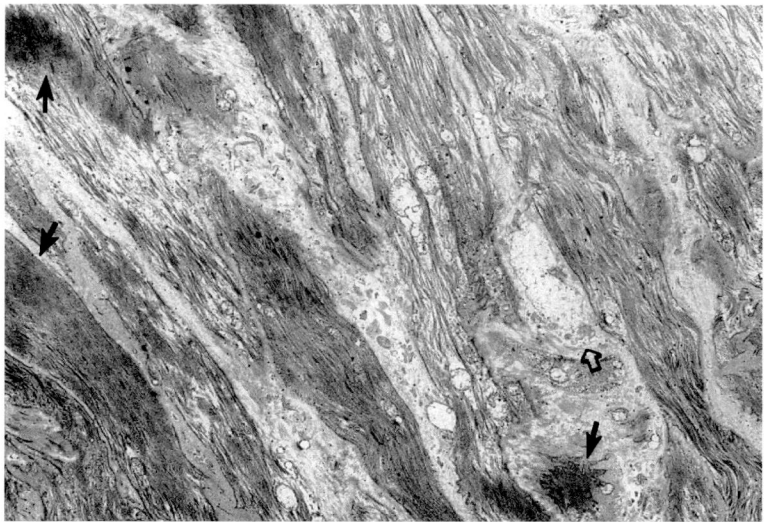

Fig. 2. Degenerating muscle cells in a detrusor with impaired bladder function due to decompensation. Myofilaments are stacked, disorganized, and disrupted (→ on the upper left) in the sarcoplasm, which is containing large vacuoles (⇒). On the right apoptosis of a muscle cell is seen (reprinted with permission, Elbadawi et al. 1993a)

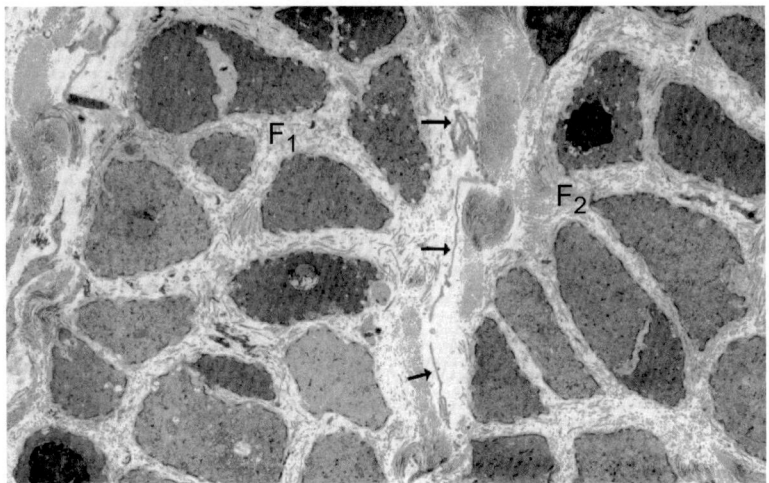

Fig. 3. Expanded intercellular spaces are seen in two muscle fascicles in an obstructed detrusor (*F1*; *F2*). The fascicles are still junctioned (→) Containing abundant fibrils plus many collagen and elastic fibres. Hypertrophic muscle cells stand out in their distinctive large and braided profiles with eccentric nuclei (reprinted with permission, Elbadawi et al. 1993b)

physiological unity of the muscle. These changes correlate with an impaired bladder contraction.

Ultrasonographic studies of the bladder show an increased diameter of the bladder wall due to an increase in connective tissue but no hypertrophy of detrusor muscle. These findings offer a theoretical explanation for high post-void residual volumes in patients with benign prostate hyperplasia after transurethral de-obstruction, even if performed by an experienced surgeon.

3.   Innervation of the bladder

The peripheral innervation of the bladder as well as spinal and associated supraspinal control mechanisms of the lower urinary tract are still not clear yet. Only few models are accepted.

3.1   Central innervation

The central control of micturition is situated in the pontocerebrum. Two regions of brain stem neurons, localised in the dorsolateral pons, are involved in the cycle of micturition. The medial M-region, known as the pontine micturition center, is the equivalent of Barrington's nucleus, which projects via long-descending pathways into the intermediolateral cell columnae, which contain autonomic motor neurons of the detrusor muscle (Fig. 4). The lateral L-region (Fig. 5), known as the pontine storage centre,

Micturition pathways

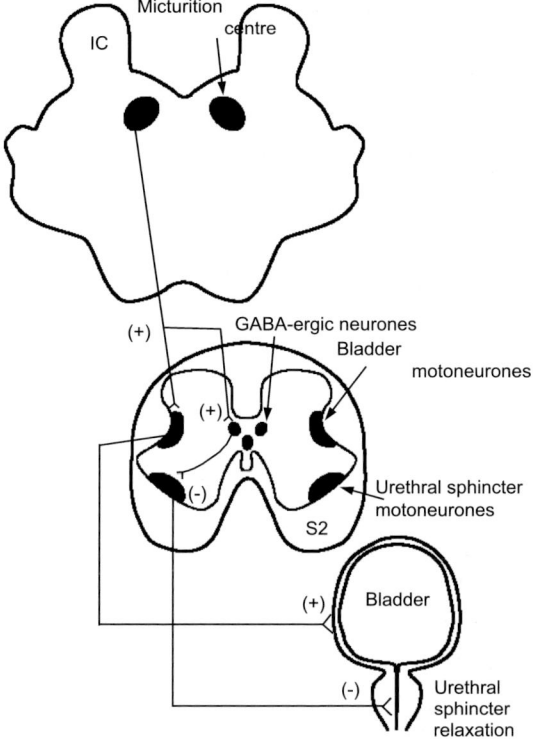

Fig. 4. Central pathways of micturition. *IC* inferior colliculus

projects throughout the spinal cord to the nucleus of Onuf, thus innervating the pelvic floor, including the external urethral sphincter (Blok et al. 1998a, 1998b; de Groat et al. 1990; Holstege et al. 1986).

In the cat, ascending projections from the sacral cord were reported to convey information on bladder filling, terminating in the periaqueductal gray (PAG) (Blok et al. 1997a). If the bladder is sufficiently filled voiding is induced by stimulating the M-region of the periaqueductal gray which results in the initiation of a normal micturition reflex. The M-region also receives afferents from the cerebral preoptic area, which might be involved in the decision when to start micturition.

In order to identify the involvement of the cerebrum during micturition, healthy, right-handed men (age range 21–50 years) were investigated by positron emission tomography (PET) (Blok et al. 1997c). Sources of activation were found in the right dorsomedial pontine tegmentum, the periaqueductal gray, the hypothalamus, and the right inferior frontal gyrus during micturition. Retention of urine was associated with a decreasing signal in the right anterior cingulate gyrus. Some of these volunteers were not able to void during the experiment. In this group, an increasing signal was recorded originating from the right ventral pontine tegmentum, an area

Urinary continence pathways

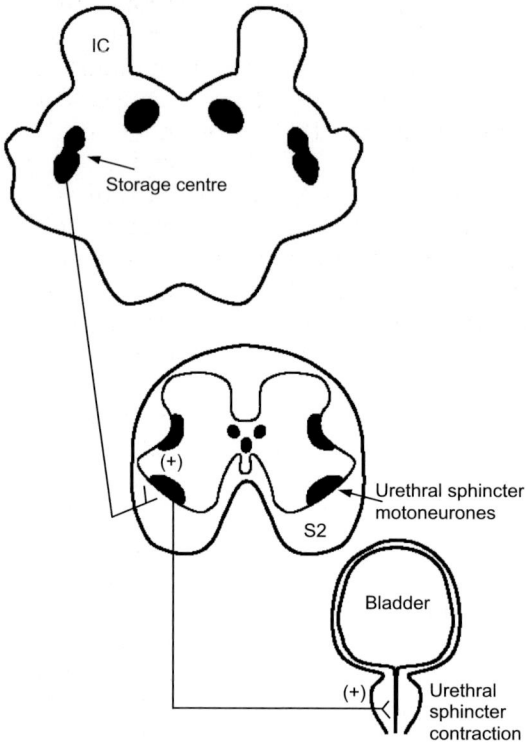

Fig. 5. Central pathways of continence. *IC* inferior colliculus

known to be associated with the control of motor neurons of the pelvic floor in the cat. Increased blood flow was also found in the right inferior frontal gyrus during unsuccessful attempts at micturition. However, little is known about the central pathways and mechanisms of supraspinal control for physiological voiding, or the reason for dysfunctional voiding, particularly in the aging population.

3.2 Age-related changes of cerebral control

The brain as a postmitotic structure is particularly vulnerable to age-related changes. Senescence is by far the most powerful risk factor for neurological diseases in elderly people, such as Alzheimer's disease or stroke (Johnson et al. 1999, Welch et al. 1998). With aging, both "normal" senescent age-related changes and late-onset diseases affect the brain, producing declines in its performance. Multiple molecular, cellular, structural, and functional changes occur in the brain during aging. Neural cells may succumb to neurodegenerative cascades resulting in disorders, such as Alzheimer's and Parkinson's disease. Morphological changes occurring in the aging brain are found particularly pronounced in neurodegenerative diseases. Systemic degenerations of selective brain areas – for example, in Parkinson or Alzheimer's disease (basal ganglia or white matter of the brain) – may be considered as models of accelerated aging. Intensive research of impaired bladder function in these diseases will result in a better understanding of the central control of micturition and possible age-related changes due to impaired bladder function (Jünemann et al. 1990, Kotkin et al. 1996, Schurch 2000). The involvement of the extrapyramidal neuronal network in the process of micturition can be seen in different studies. Stimulation of the globus pallidum and other extrapyramidal structures inhibits voiding (Lewin et al. 1965, 1967), whereas stereotactic thalamotomia results in detrusor activation (Murdock et al. 1975). First results of deep brain-stimulated patients with Parkinson's disease reported decreased detrusor hypersensibility and an increasing capacity of the urinary bladder owing to a more physiological situation (Seif et al. 2003).

In patients with and without dementia complaining of urge incontinence, anticholinergic medication led to an increasing bladder capacity although subjective improvement was only observed in patients without dementia (Sugiyama et al. 1993). It was suggested that the major cause of incontinence in elderly patients was not an impaired cerebral control of micturition but the specific conditions of demented patients such as agnosia and apraxia. Additionally, failure of the bladder reflex has been hypothesized as another component of lower urinary tract symptoms in aging male and female. Patients recognise they are occasionally incapable to anticipate when a bladder contraction may occur (McGuire 1994). Investigations involving the use of functional magnet resonance tomography may be helpful for investigation of cortical and subcortical mechanisms during micturition in healthy and incontinent elderly people. This may add important information concerning physiological processes and consequences of cerebral ageing.

At the cellular and molecular level, multiple mechanisms are known to maintain the integrity of nerve cell circuits, facilitate responses to environmental demands, and promote recovery of function after injury. Aging of the brain can be facilitated by activating a hormesis response, in which neurons increase their production of neurotrophic factors and stress proteins. The neural stem cells residing in the adult brain are also responsive to environmental demands and seem capable of replacing lost or dysfunctional neurons and glial cells, perhaps even in the aging brain. Recent application of modern methods of molecular and cellular biology to the problem of brain aging has shown remarkable capacity of brain cells to adapt during aging and resist development of diseases (Mattson et al. 2002). Further research will have to show how these hopeful results can be used to preserve bladder innervation and thus prevent incontinence in elderly patients.

3.3   Peripheral innervation

The nerve supply to the urinary bladder is both sympathetic and parasympathetic. The sympathetic innervation originates from Th_{11-12}

and L_{1-2} levels of the spinal cord and eventually becomes part of the hypogastric plexus continuing on to the bladder and urethra. β-adrenergic innervation of the bladder allows the detrusor muscle to accommodate during filling.

The extrinsic urethral sphincter as well as the levator ani and the pelvic floor are innervated by somatic nerve fibres that emanate from sacral roots S_2 and S_3 (De Araujo et al. 1982). Autonomic nerve branches originate from S_2–S_4 to form the pelvic plexus that is innervating the detrusor muscle and the smooth musculature of the urethra. However, there are a few somatic nerve branches emanating from S_2 and S_3 that run close to the levator ani muscle and the external rhabdosphincter around the membranous urethra. Topographically, these nerve fibres run on the inner side of the levator ani muscle caudal to the striated periurethral sling to innervate one component of the external sphincter. Another contribution to the urinary continence mechanism derives from the pudendal nerve that innervates the pelvic floor, especially the transversus perinei muscle. The pudendal nerve is part of the sacral plexus and formed by somatic components of S_2–S_4 nerve roots once they combine to one major nerve trunk superior to the coccygeus muscle (Jünemann et al. 1988). The neural contribution of each neuromuscular component to the external urethral closure pressure was determined by selective neurostimulation of S_2, S_3 and the pudendal nerve (Jünemann et al. 1988). Prior to and after selective neurotomy or xylocaine blockade it was convincingly shown that somatic fibres of S_2 innervate the transversus perinei muscle, whereas fibres from S_3 control the intrinsic urethral rhabdosphincter and levator ani muscle (Jünemann et al. 1988). However, both nerval segments demonstrated a crossing over in the innervation of the other sphincter components. The pudendal nerve runs anterior to the coccygeal muscle through the pars infrapiriforme of the foramen ischiadicum, then passes through the foramen ischiadicum minus into the canalis pudendalis (Alcok's canal) and divides into the rectal nerves, perineal nerves, and the dorsal penile nerve or dorsal clitoral nerve respectively (Jünemann et al. 1987, Rauber et al. 1988).

Autonomic nerve fibres are connected to afferent and efferent fibres of somatic nerves – for example the mixed somatomotoric pudendal nerve arise from the sacral spinal cord (S_1–S_3). Afferent nociceptive or proprioceptive information, conducted by the pudendal nerve from the external urethra sphincter, may modulate the detrusor function. Neuromodulation of the lower urinary tract by peripheral electrical stimulation of different somatic afferents, as well as neuromodulation of sacral spinal nerves has been described for the treatment of dysfunctional voiding and neurogenic bladder symptoms (Schmidt et al. 1978; Tanagho et al. 1982, 1992, 1988; Braun et al. 1999).

A close proximity of the sacral plexus to the ureter were reported in cadaveric studies (Leissner et al. 2001). Single fibres reaching out of the pelvic plexus were located about 1.5 cm dorsal and medial to the ureterovesical junction. The bundles of the pelvic plexus terminated at the distal ureter, trigone, and rectum.

Unilateral denervation of the detrusor muscle results from injury of the pelvic plexus. Jünemann et al. reported the unilateral innervation via the plexus pelvicus to the trigonum vesicae in electrophysiological studies (Jünemann et al. 2001b). A strict unilateral stimulation of the plexus pelvicus in the animal model (Göttinger mini-pig) showed a contraction of the detrusor only on the stimulated side. The risk of surgical procedures increases with age, and these findings should be considered when dealing with patients with dysfunctional voiding and a history of pelvic surgery.

4.   Pathophysiology

The normal function of the bladder during filling and voiding can be assessed by urodynamics and video cystometry.

4.1   Physiology of the filling phase

With increasing filling of the bladder, the detrusor expands so that the intravesical pressure rises only minimally to 20 cm H_2O at maximal capacity. This process happens nearly unnoticed since afferent signals are subject to both spinal and cerebral suppression. A first subjective impression of a filled bladder arises from a volume of 150–250 ml upwards; when the maximum bladder capacity of 350–450 ml is reached, it is perceived as urinary urge. By means of deliberate inhibition of the micturition reflex, the detrusor contraction can be suppressed until the external conditions allow an emptying of the bladder. During storage phase, the bladder remains tightly closed, while the activity of the external urethral sphincter increases gradually. The increase in intra-abdominal and intravesical pressure is compensated through a reflex-induced increase in muscle activity, which is, in turn, triggered by a pressure increase in the urethra. Thus, the closure pressure of the urethra is always higher than the intravesical pressure, which guarantees continence both in neutral and in stress situations.

4.2   Physiology of micturition

Micturition is initiated by deliberate activation of the micturition reflex. The cerebral inhibitory impulses on the sacral micturition centre are replaced by stimulating efferences. During the filling of the bladder, the L-region of pontocerebrum is activated to increase the tonus of the external urethral sphincter. When the functional bladder capacity reaches its maximum, the afferent information is conducted via the spinal cord to the periaquaeductal gray. Now the M-region on the pontocerebrum excites the neural structures and initiates voiding by stimulating the detrusor muscle and relaxing the musculus sphincter externus. During this process, intravesical pressure exceeds the closure pressure of the urethra. This synergic interaction of urethral relaxation and detrusor contraction results in a strong urinary flow and emptying of the bladder without residual urine.

A deliberate interruption of micturition through contraction of the musculus sphincter externus is accompanied by a reflex-induced intermission of detrusor contraction. This coordination of storage and voiding is under both cerebral and spinal control. Keeping this in mind it is obvious that a young child, whose efferent nerve pathways are still immature and who has yet to be conditioned by a learning process, has no control over its voiding function. Again, this is the reason why paraplegics with spinal damage above the sacral micturition centre are incontinent owing to failure of the central control mechanisms; another example are patients with dementia, cerebral-sclerotic or neurological diseases voiding in an uncontrolled manner.

So far, it is not yet clear, which central, neuronal, structural, and functional changes are responsible for impairing the physiological micturition process with aging, when they begin to occur, and which functional consequences result. Future investigation will be necessary, to search for appropriate therapeutic measures for tackling the problem of age-related incontinence effectively.

4.3   Pathophysiology of the aging bladder in subvesical outflow obstruction

The functional capacity of the urinary bladder is the terminate to initiate voiding; it is lower than the absolute capacity theoretically achieved by passive filling during anaesthesia. Figure 6 shows the correlation between intravesical pressure and actual bladder filling during contraction. Kaplan et al. demonstrated that the intravesical pressure is higher at lower intravesical volumes but may be sustained only for a shorter period (Kaplan et al. 1991). Therefore an optimal relation has to exist between intravesical bladder volume and energy input. If only small micturition volumes are reached before the initiation of the micturition reflex, all symptoms of urgency with or without incontinence or increasing voiding frequency will occur. However, if intravesical volume is too high, the bladder cannot be emptied completely, resulting in increased residual volumes after voiding.

The bladder capacity changes with age and depends on physiological circumstances. The two main variables affecting the bladder capacity are distension of the detrusor muscle and the interval between voiding attempts. Particularly in elderly patients both parameters may be affected. Repeated voiding to improve emptying is traditionally recommended to patients with increased residual urine volumes, and distension of the bladder is commonly caused by subvesical outflow obstruction associated with prostate hypertrophy or sclerosis of the bladder neck.

Bross et al. investigated the effect of double voiding in an animal model (Bross et al. 1999a). In four series with different intervals between consecutive stimulations (1 min, 3 min, 5 min, 15 min), the maximum intravesical pressure was measured during each stimulation. It was shown that the detrusor pressure was nearly 100% when the interval between the two incidences of sacral neurostimulation inducing bladder contraction was

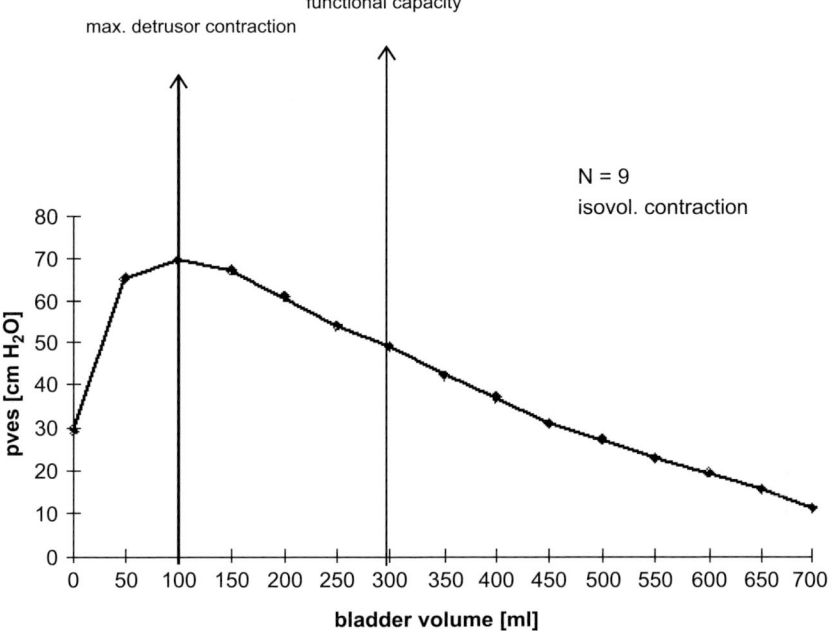

Fig. 6. Detrusor pressure when stimulating at different filling volumes in 9 foxhounds (reprinted with permission; Bross et al. 1999b)

30 min. By reducing the interval, a decreasing attainable maximum of intravesical pressure during the second contraction was observed. An interval of five minutes reduced the pressure stepwise, and after five contractions the pressure reached only 90% of the pressure compared to the initial response. By reducing the interval to 3 min and finally to 1 min, values of only 70–80% were achieved (Fig. 7).

This model has not been tested in humans, but it raises an important question. It may be counterproductive to recommend the procedure of double voiding, for example, in patients with chronic subvesical outflow obstruction. It may in fact serve to further impairment of bladder function instead of lowering post voiding residual volumes. Further studies, especially in elderly patients, are necessary to examine the importance of the time interval between voiding attempts.

Bladder distension, either acute or chronic, is another common event in aging patients. Most commonly, it is caused by outflow obstruction combined with decreased bladder sensation and an inability to perceive increasing post-void residual volumes, which indicates an altered central assimilation of the sensory input, especially in the bladder of elderly people.

A correlation between bladder filling volume and detrusor pressure during contraction after sacral (S_2, S_3) anterior root stimulation in the male foxhound was recently reported (Bross et al. 1999b). While bladder volumes were continuously increased from 50 ml to 700 ml (the latter representing overdistension), the maximum attainable detrusor pressures during contrac-

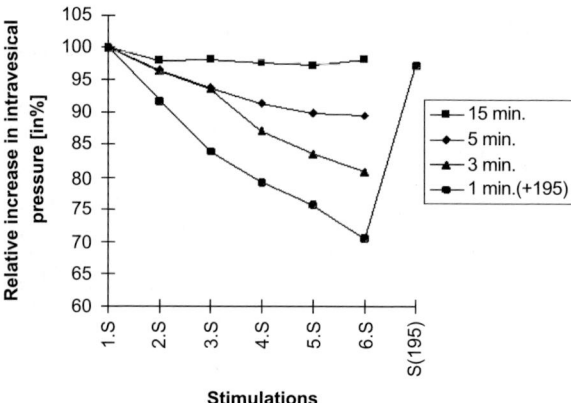

Fig. 7. Repetitive stimulation of the detrusor. A decreasing intravesical pressure results from reducing the interval of stimulation (reprinted with permission; Bross et al. 1999a)

tion decreased. Repeated bladder filling in the same way 15 minutes after overdistension resulted in a further reduction of maximum bladder pressure by almost 28% (Figs. 8, 9). If a single overdistension can lead to detrusor decompensation, it must be prevented to preserve an adequate motor function of the bladder. In patients with subvesical obstruction, active intravesical pressure never suffices for adequate micturition during over-distention. This explains the fact that the detrusor can decompensate after large fluid intake, resulting in urinary retention. Without emptying the bladder, for example by catheterisation, this results in a vicious circle with bladder overdistention, overflow incontinence, and partially irreversible damage of the detrusor. In addition to these clinical findings, ultrastructural investigations of the detrusor after overdistension observed nerve degenerations such as axonal swelling and lysis of cell organelles (Sehn 1979, Tammela et al. 1987). Lasanen et al. showed that detrusor overdistention resulted in cholinergic hypo-innervation, which was already observed 7 days after the distension, persisting up to 21 days (Lasanen et al. 1992). Afterwards, the cholinergic nerves were then completely recovered. These results have to be reproduced in the human model, especially in elderly patients.

Are there parameters concerning the functional quality of the chronically obstructed detrusor muscle? Can we predict postoperative post-void residual volumes? When should surgery be recommended for de-obstruction, especially in the old multimorbid patient? A typical urodynamic finding in subvesical outflow obstruction is the high pressure required for bladder emptying, with a decreasing urinary flow during voiding. This could be the result of increasing resistance due to benign prostate hyperplasia or contraction of the bladder neck, resulting in inadequate bladder emptying and high posturinary bladder volume. If there is an abnormally increased pressure during voiding, the bladder should be de-obstructed. In patients with pathologically increased pressures of $60\,cm/H_2O$ and more during

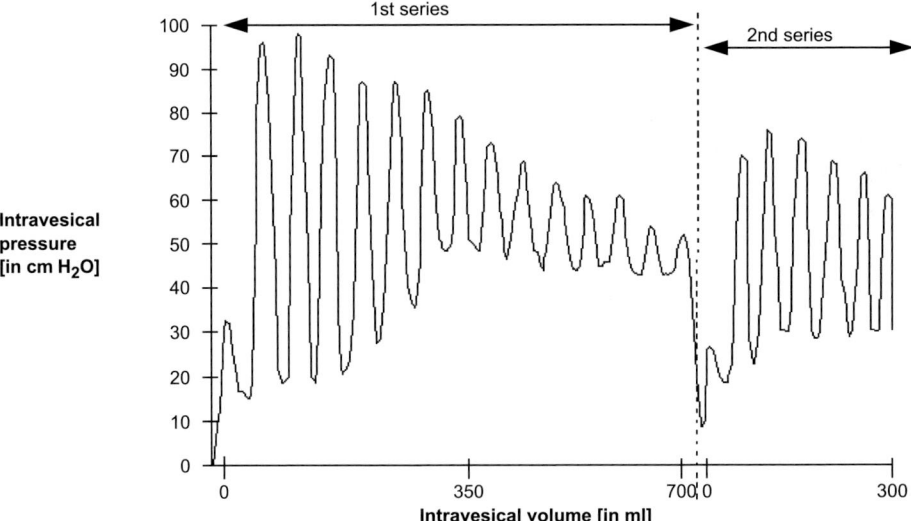

Fig. 8. The original measurement of the intravesical pressure is demonstrated in 1 dog. On the left side, the first series up to 700 ml is shown and the second series on the right side. In both series, the bladder response was influenced by the intravesical volume. Maximum pressure was observed at 100 ml. After overdistention, a reduction in maximum pressure of 28,6% was seen (reprinted with permission; Bross et al. 1999b)

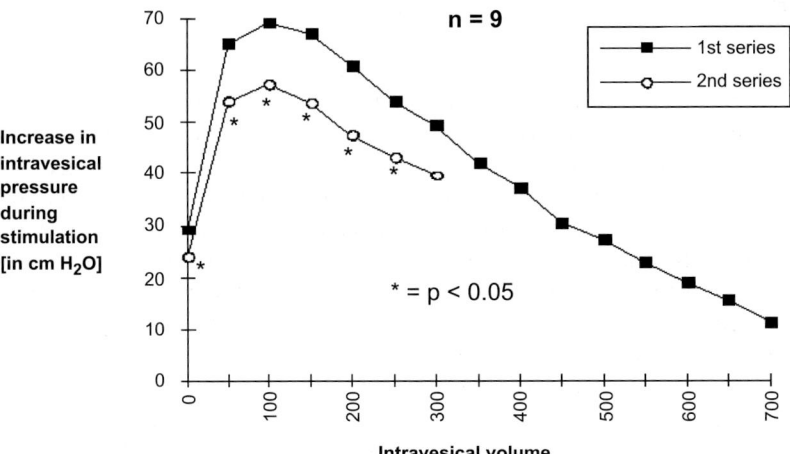

Fig. 9. Mean increase in intravesical pressure during stimulation is demonstrated in 9 foxhounds. The bladder response was significantly reduced during overdistention ($p < 0.01$ at 700 ml) compared with maximum pressure at 100 ml. After overdistention, the bladder response was significantly reduced at 0–250 ml ($p < 0.05$) (reprinted with permission; Bross et al. 1999b)

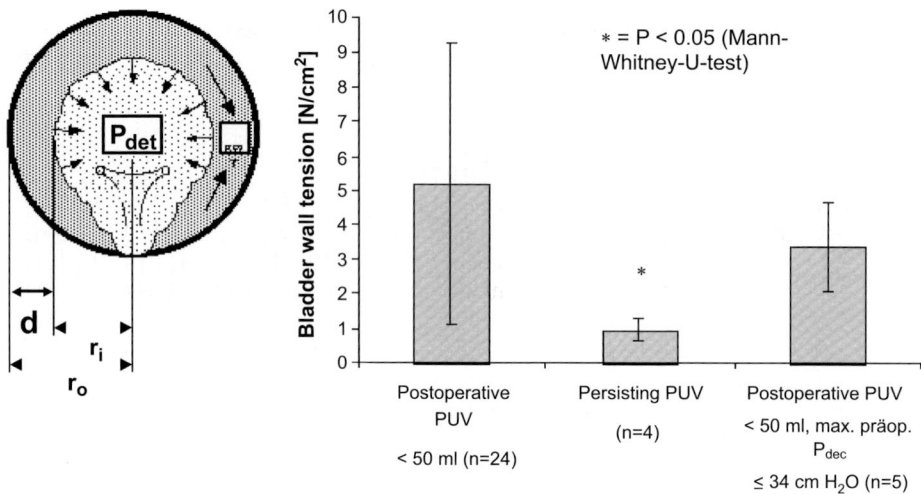

Fig. 10. Left: Bladder wall tension (BWT) calculated by formula based on force keeping 2 hemispheres together. Determining detrusor pressure, radius and bladder wall thickness is necessary for calculation. *BWT* Bladder wall tension (in N/cm^2); *Pdet* detrusor pressure (in cm H$_2$O) $\times$ 0,97969 $\times$ 10^{-2}; r_i inner radius (in cm); r_o external radius (in cm); *d* bladder wall thickness (in cm). Right: Bladder wall tension as predictive value to post-void residual urine (PUV) after subvesical de-obstruction (reprinted with permission; Bross et al. 2001)

voiding, non-significant postoperative post-void residual volumes can be observed. But in patients with LUTS and a non-obstructive detrusor pressure profile during voiding, an average of post-void residual volumes of 150–200 ml after transurethral de-obstruction can be measured. However, some patients with non-obstructive, normal detrusor pressure profile do not experience postoperative post-void residual. Detrusor pressure alone is therefore an unreliable predictor of post-void residual urine after surgery. Recent investigations may gain predictive value. Bross et al. reported on detrusor wall tension as a predictive parameter for post-void residual volumes by evaluating both bladder wall thickness and detrusor wall tension (Bross et al. 2001). Patients with increased detrusor wall tension had no increase in postoperative post void residual volumes, whereas patients with decreased tension of the detrusor wall experienced postoperative post-void residual volume (Fig. 10).

5.   Conclusion

The bladder is exposed to a variety of influences during aging. The central control of micturition and coordination of the lower urinary tract plays an important role in the development of age-related dysfunctions. Further research is needed to improve the knowledge of these central mechanisms and their pathophysiology to protect elderly patients from increasing negative consequences to health and social life.

6.   References

1. Blok BF, Holstege G (1997a) Ultrastructural evidence for a direct pathway from the pontine micturition center to the parasympathetic preganglionic motoneurons of the bladder of the cat. Neurosci Lett 222: 195–198
2. Blok BF, Holstege G (1998a) The central nervous system control of micturition in cats and humans. Behav Brain Res 92: 119–125
3. Blok BF, Holstege G (1998b) Brain activation during micturition in women. Brain 121: 2033–2042
4. Blok BF, Sturms LM, Holstege G (1997b) A PET study on cortical and subcortical control of pelvic floor musculature in women. J Comp Neurol 389: 535–544
5. Blok BF, Willemsen AT, Holstege G (1997c) A PET study on brain control of micturition in humans. Brain 120: 111–121
6. Braun PM, Boschert J, Bross S, Scheepe JR, Alken P, Jünemann KP (1999) Tailored laminectomy: a new technique for neuromodulator implantation. J Urol 162: 1607–1609
7. Bross S, Schumacher S, Scheepe JR, Braun PM, Alken P, Jünemann KP (2001) Combined evaluation of detrusor pressure and bladder wall thickness as a parameter for the assessment of detrusor function: an experimental in vivo study. J Urol 166: 1130–1135
8. Bross S, Schumacher S, Scheepe JR, Seif C, Jünemann KP, Alken P (1999a) Smooth muscle fatigue due to repeated urinary bladder neurostimulation: an in vivo study. Neurourol Urodyn 18: 41–53
9. Bross S, Schumacher S, Scheepe JR, Zendler S, Braun PM, Alken P, Jünemann KP (1999b) Effects of acute urinary bladder overdistension on bladder response during sacral neurostimulation. Eur Urol 36: 354–359
10. DeAraujo CG, Schmidt RA, Tanagho EA (1982) Neural pathway to the lower urinary tract identified by retrograde axonal transport of horseradish peroxidase. Urology 19: 290–295
11. deGroat WC, Steers WD (1990) Autonomic regulation of the urinary bladder and sex organs. In: Loewy AD, SKM (eds) Central regulation of autonomic function. University Press Oxford: Oxford, pp 310–333
12. Dixon J, Gosling J (1987) Structure and innervation in the human. In: Torrens M, Morrison J (eds) The physiology of the lower urinary tract. Springer: Berlin, Heidelberg, New York, Tokyo, pp 1–22
13. Dorschner W, Stolzenburg JU, Neuhaus J (2001) Anatomic principles of urinary incontinence. Urologe A 40: 223–233
14. Elbadawi A, Diokno AC, Millard RJ (1998) The aging bladder: morphology and urodynamics. World J Urol 16: S10–S34
15. Elbadawi A, Hailemariam S, Yalla SV, Resnick NM (1997) Structural basis of geriatric voiding dysfunction. VII. Prospective ultrastructural/urodynamic evaluation of its natural evolution. J Urol 157: 1814–1822
16. Elbadawi A, Yalla SV, Resnick NM (1993a) Structural basis of geriatric voiding dysfunction. II. Aging detrusor: normal versus impaired contractility. J Urol 150: 1657–1667
17. Elbadawi A, Yalla SV, Resnick NM (1993b) Structural basis of geriatric voiding dysfunction. IV. Bladder outlet obstruction. J Urol 150: 1681–1695

18. Hextall A, Bidmead J, Cardozo L, Hooper R (2001a) The impact of the menstrual cycle on urinary symptoms and the results of urodynamic investigation. BJOG 108: 1193–1196

19. Hextall A, Cardozo L (2001b) The role of estrogen supplementation in lower urinary tract dysfunction. Int Urogynecol J Pelvic Floor Dysfunct 12: 258–261

20. Hinman F (1993) Atlas of urosurgical anatomy. Saunders: Philadelphia, pp 334–338

21. Holstege G, Griffiths D, deWall H, Dalm E (1986) Anatomical and physiological observations on supraspinal control of bladder and urethral sphincter muscles in the cat. J Comp Neurol 250: 449–461

22. Hutch JA (1967) A new theory of the anatomy of the internal urinary sphincter and the physiology of micturition. V. The base plate and stress incontinence. Obstet Gynecol 30: 309–317

23. Jackson SR, Avery NC, Tarlton JF, Eckford SD, Abrams P, Bailey AJ (1996) Changes in metabolism of collagen in genitourinary prolapse. Lancet 347: 1658–1661

24. Johnson FB, Sinclair DA, Guarente L (1999) Molecular biology of aging. Cell 96: 291–302

25. Jünemann KP (2000) Therapeutische Optionen der Altersinkontinenz. In: Jocham D, Altwein J, Jünemann KP, Schmitz-Draeger BJ, Weidner W, Wirth M (eds) Aging Male Man(n) wird nicht jünger. Verlag im Kilian: Marburg, pp 63–71

26. Jünemann KP (2001a) Comment on the contribution by Dorschner W, Neuhaus J, Stolzenburg JU. Anatomic principles of urinary incontinence. Urologe A 40: 237–238

27. Jünemann KP, Lue TF, Schmidt RA, Tanagho EA (1988) Clinical significance of sacral and pudendal nerve anatomy. J Urol 139: 74–80

28. Jünemann KP, Martinez Portillo FJ, Seif C, Braun PM, Leissner J, Hohenfellner R (2001b) Risiko der Detrusordenervation bei Antirefluxchirurgie verdeutlicht am neurophysiologischen Modell. Urologe A 40 (1) [Suppl]: 64

29. Jünemann KP, Melchior H (1990) Disorders of bladder function in Parkinson syndrome. Urologe A 29: 170–175

30. Jünemann KP, Schmidt RA, Melchior H, Tanagho EA (1987) Neuroanatomy and clinical significance of the external urethral sphincter. Urol Int 42: 132–136

31. Kotkin L, Milam DF (1996) Evaluation and management of the urologic consequences of neurologic disease. Tech Urol 2: 210–219

32. Lasanen LT, Tammela TL, Kallioinen M, Waris T (1992) Effect of acute distension on cholinergic innervation of the rat urinary bladder. Urol Res 20: 59–62

33. Leissner J, Allhoff EP, Wolff W, Feja C, Hockel M, Black P, Hohenfellner R (2001) The pelvic plexus and antireflux surgery: topographical findings and clinical consequences. J Urol 165: 1652–1655

34. Lewin RJ, Dillard GV, Porter RW (1967) Extrapyramidal inhibition of the urinary bladder. Brain Res 4: 301–307

35. Lewin RJ, Porter RW (1965) Inhibition of spontaneous bladder activity by stimulation of the globus pallidus. Neurology 15: 1049–1052

36. Maggi C (1993) Nervous control of the urogenital system. In: Maggi CA (ed) Autonomic nervous system – Physiology. Harwood Academic Publishing: Chur, Schweiz, pp 3

37. Mattson MP, Chan SL, Duan W (2002) Modification of brain aging and neurodegenerative disorders by genes, diet, and behavior. Physiol Rev 82: 637–672

38. McGuire EJ (1994) Idiopathic bladder instability. In: Kursh ED, McGuire EJ (eds) Female Urology. Philadelphia: Lippincott, pp 95–101
39. Melchior H (1995) Disorders of bladder function in the elderly. Urologe A 34: 329–333
40. Moore KN (1999) A review of the anatomy of the male continence mechanism and the cause of urinary incontinence after prostatectomy. J Wound Ostomy Continence Nurs 26: 86–93
41. Murdock MI, Olsson CA, Sax DS, Krane RJ (1975) Effects of levodopa on the bladder outlet. J Urol 113: 803–805
42. Myers RP, Goellner JR, Cahill DR (1987) Prostate shape, external striated urethral sphincter and radical prostatectomy: the apical dissection. J Urol 138: 543–550
43. Petros PE, Ulmsten UI (1990) An integral theory of female urinary incontinence. Experimental and clinical considerations. Acta Obstet Gynecol Scand [Suppl] 153: 7–31
44. Rauber A, Kopsch F (1988) Topographie der Organsysteme, Systematik der peripheren Leitungsbahnen. Thieme: New York
45. Schmidt RA, Bruschini H, Tanagho EA (1978) Feasibility of inducing micturition through chronic stimulation of sacral roots. Urology 7: 471–477
46. Schreiter F, Fuchs P, Stockamp K (1976) Estrogenic sensitivity of alpha-receptors in the urethra musculature. Urol Int 31: 13–19
47. Schurch B (2000) Neurogenic voiding disorders. Current status of diagnosis and therapy. Schweiz Med Wochenschr 130: 1618–1626
48. Sehn JT (1979) The ultrastructural effect of distension on the neuromuscular apparatus of the urinary bladder. Invest Urol 16: 369–375
49. Seif C, Herzog J, van der Horst C, Volkmann J, Deuschl G, Jünemann KP, Braun PM (2003) Impact of STN stimulation on the bladder function in patients with idiopathic Parkinson syndrome. Ann Neurol (in press)
50. Smith AR, Hosker GL, Warrell DW (1989a) The role of partial denervation of the pelvic floor in the aetiology of genitourinary prolapse and stress incontinence of urine. A neurophysiological study. Br J Obstet Gynaecol 96: 24–28
51. Smith AR, Hosker GL, Warrell DW (1989b) The role of pudendal nerve damage in the aetiology of genuine stress incontinence in women. Br J Obstet Gynaecol 96: 29–32
52. Snooks SJ, Swash M (1984a) Abnormalities of the innervation of the urethral striated sphincter musculature in incontinence. Br J Urol 56: 401–405
53. Snooks SJ, Swash M, Setchell M, Henry MM (1984b) Injury to innervation of pelvic floor sphincter musculature in childbirth. Lancet 8: 546–550
54. Strasser H, Klima G, Poisel S, Horninger W, Bartsch G (1996) Anatomy and innervation of the rhabdosphincter of the male urethra. Prostate 28: 24–31
55. Sugiyama T, Matsuda H, Oonishi N, Kiwamoto H, Esa A, Park YC, Kurita T, Uchida A, Kunikata S (1993) Anticholinergic therapy of urinary incontinence and urinary frequency associated with the elderly-with special reference to dementia. Nippon Hinyokika Gakkai Zasshi 84: 1068–1073
56. Tammela T, Autio-Harmainen H, Lukkarinen O, Sormunen R (1987) Effect of distension on function and nervous ultrastructure in the canine urinary bladder. Urol Int 42: 265–270
57. Tanagho EA, Schmidt RA (1982) Bladder pacemaker: scientific basis and clinical future. Urology 20: 614–619
58. Tanagho EA, Schmidt RA (1988) Electrical stimulation in the clinical management of neurogenic bladder. J Urol 140: 1331–1339

59. Tanagho EA, Smith DR (1966) The anatomy and function of the bladder neck. Br J Urol 38: 54–71
60. Tanagho EA (1992) Anatomy of the lower urinay tract. In: Walsh PC, Retik AB, Stamey TA, Vaughn ED (eds) Campbell's urology. Saunders: Philadelphia, pp 40–45
61. Welch WJ, Gambetti P (1998) Chaperoning brain diseases. Nature 392: 23–24

Correspondence address: Christof van der Horst, MD, Department of Urology, University of Schleswig-Holstein – Campus Kiel, Arnold-Heller-Strasse 7, D-24105 Kiel, Germany (E-mail: cvanderhorst@urology.uni-kiel.de).

Epidemiology and symptomatology of the aging bladder

L. K. Daha and *E. Plas*

Department of Urology and LBI for Urology & Andrology,
Lainz Hospital, Vienna, Austria

Contents

1.   Introduction

Life expectancy is increasing worldwide, with an estimated expectancy at birth of 78 years in Western Europe, 76 years in North America, 69 years in Latin America and the Caribbean, 65 years in Asia, and 49 years in Sub-Saharan Africa. Prolongation of life expectancy was achieved by reduction of infant death and medical progress in treating chronic disorders. This has resulted not only in an increase in numbers but also in proportions of older persons. It is estimated that worldwide proportion of persons older than 65 years will more than double from 6.9% to 16.4% between 2000 and 2050. In the next 25 years, the population aged 65 and above is likely to grow by 88% compared with an increase of only 45% in the working age population. Additionally, the proportion of people above 80 years will increase from 1.9% to 4.2%, with an estimated increase of over 100 year old people from 135 000 in 1998 to 2.2 million in 2050, a more than 16-fold increase. This trend has been consistent in several countries, for example, 32% of Austria's population will be older than 60 by 2030.

However, differences in life expectancy between the richest and poorest countries still remain. The annual report of the United Nation Development Programme (UNDP) 1997 reported on a wide range between developing countries (4% population older than 65 years) compared with industrialised countries (13% older than 65 years). Additionally, life expectancy of women remains 5–8 years higher compared with men, leading to a female:male ratio of the oldest-old of 4:1 (World Health Organization Aging and Life Course 2001).

The constant increase in the world's population and the proportions of elderly people confront society with new, emerging problems including social, political, and economic issues. One major aspect is aging and health, creating a new segment in medicine to establish healthy aging. Health has been defined by the WHO as "a state of complete physical, mental and social well-being and not merely the absence of diseases or infirmity". It should be maintained throughout life to achieve "an acceptable quality of life in older individuals and to ensure continued contributions of older persons to society" (World Health Organization Aging and Life Course 2001). But the process of aging is influenced by several factors including the environment, society, the economy, lifestyle, and sex, cultural, and spiritual determinants.

Considering only health issues, aging is associated with increasing comorbidity of several organ systems including metabolic, cardiovascular (Fig. 1), intestinal, neurological, endocrine, orthopaedic, and, last but not less important, urogenital disorders. These diseases have a significant impact not only on patients but also on healthcare budgets with increasing costs, since 90% of medications are prescribed in the last 10 years of life.

In addition to that, disease- and age related consultations in hospitals change with increasing life expectancy. We reported on the characteristics

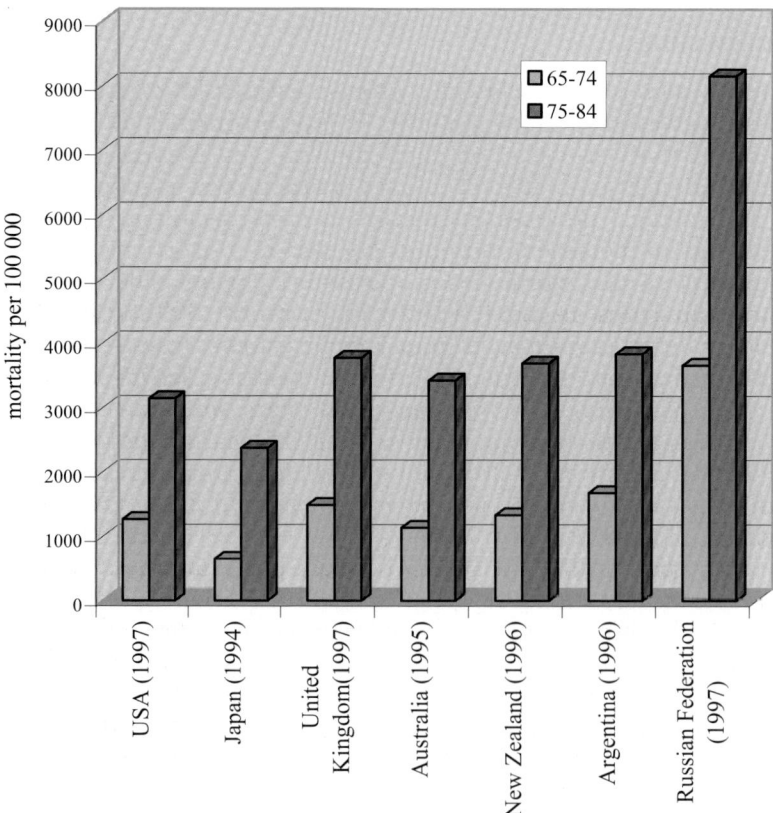

Fig. 1. Cardiovascular specific mortality (per 100 000) in different continents (WHO)

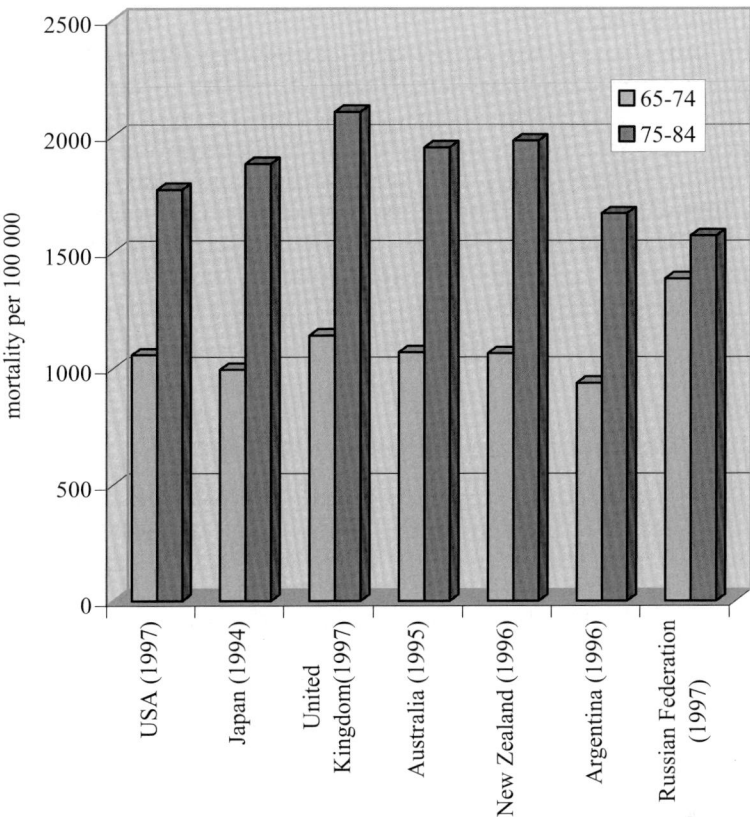

Fig. 2. Cancer specific mortality (per 100 000) in different continents (WHO)

of patients attending our in- and outpatient clinic in 1996 and 1997, representing a urological department in a large community hospital with 1200 beds and an affiliated nursing care home centre with 3500 beds (Daha et al. 2002). 36% of patients requiring admission to hospital and 58% attending our outpatient clinic were older than 60 years. 10% of patients requiring admission to hospital were older than 80 years.

The triangle of increased life expectancy, comorbidity, and costs confronts society with new problems. Higher incidence of diseases and comorbidity in the aging population requires special programs for prevention and treatment. But the issue of healthy aging concerns not only patients but families, society, the economy, and healthcare budgets. Chronic diseases often require observations in nursing homes. In 1990, half a million Austrians required extramural nursing care (Badelt et al. 1996). Extrapolating this to the year 2030 results in an estimated 800,000 people requiring some form of nursing care. If preventive activities are successful this may decrease to 645,000, accompanied by significant savings in health expenses. However, the need for nursing homes for people of increasing age will be reduced not only by preventing the main causes of death, such as cardiovascular disease and cancer (Olshansky et al. 1991). It will be necessary to establish not only therapeutic but also social and political strategies to prevent rising comorbidity during aging to support healthy aging. Health awareness has become a major issue in industrialised societies. Prevention of diseases is and will remain of special interest in the future. But prevention can only be achieved over a longer period and usually does not solve current medical issues. Further, people have to be motivated to consume preventive medical care. An Austrian survey showed that less than 10% of the population took advantage of freely available, annual preventive medical checkups, including only 4.7% of men older than 75 years (Schmeiser-Rieder and Kunze 1999).

2. Incidence and prevalence of urogenital aging

The aging process is reflected in alterations of all organ systems including the genitourinary tract. The incidence of urogenital pathologies has been shown to increase with age. Between 50–69 years, the risk of genitourinary complaints in women is approximately 8–9-fold higher compared with adolescents. This again doubles in people older than 70 years (Carbone et al. 2001). Consistent with that, men in their 60s have a 25-fold higher risk of developing genitourinary disorders than men aged 20. However, this number increases again 40-fold in elderly men above 70 years. In 2001, the WHO report on men, aging and health reported benign prostatic enlargement, urinary incontinence, erectile dysfunction, and prostate cancer as the most common chronic urogenital disorders (World Health Organization Aging and Life Course 2001).

One major issue in the aging population affecting both men and women is urinary incontinence which often causes distressing symptoms. It is one of the top 10 chronic health conditions with a prevalence of 3–53% in people older than 60 years (Romanzi 2001, Tseng et al. 2000, Butler et al. 1999, Koyama et al. 1998, Stewart et al. 2002, Langa et al. 2002, Resnick 1987, Busby-Whitehead and Johnson 1998, Campbell et al. 1985, Hampel et al. 1997). Interestingly, many accept the infirmities associated with age including their genitourinary symptoms as a natural process and do not seek treatment and relief. Although the prevalence and incidence of incontinence in the aging population are high, rising comorbidity of other diseases directly affects incontinence in aging population (Welz-Barth et al. 2000). Multimorbidity was found to be the most important factor for development of distressing symptoms of the aging bladder. An increase in comorbidities correlated positively with the incidence of incontinence. Patients with five or more chronic diseases had a 100% risk of incontinence (Welz-Barth et al. 2000). This again shows the close correlation and interaction not only of the aging process of the genitourinary tract alone but also its influence on other processes such as internal diseases, hormonal alterations, obesity, and metabolic and orthopaedic disorders.

The predominant symptoms of the aging bladder are frequency, urgency, dysuria, bladder outlet obstruction, nocturia, incontinence, and recurrent urinary tract infections.

Recently, prevalence and severity of lower urinary tract symptoms in Japanese men and women were reported (Kakizaki et al. 2002). A significant age-related increase in IPSS and quality-of-life score was observed in both men and women. The percentage of urinary symptoms increased in aging men from 52% to 72% and 80% in the group of men aged 50, 60, and 70 years. This was different to women in the same age groups, who complained of incontinence in 27%, 36%, and 55% of cases. Men complained more often of voiding symptoms than women by the age of 50 and older. But, incontinence is not the only problem of the aging bladder, as shown by Barlow et al. (1997). In a large survey of more than 3000 European women aged 55–75 years from six countries, urogenital symptoms were reported by nearly 30%, with mild symptoms in up to 65% and severe symptoms in 16.5%. Urinary frequency was most frequently present in 12.7% followed by dysuria in 8.3% and incontinence in 7.4% (Knutson et al. 2001). Dysuria, frequency, and incontinence increased with aging. As the prevalence of frequency and urgency increase with aging, the incidence of genuine stress incontinence decreases annually from 0.55% to 0.43% in women in their 40s compared with their late 50s. Contrary to that, urge incontinence increases from 0.08% to 0.2% per year (Hampel et al. 1997).

Although age-related changes of bladder morphology and function occur in both men and women and expose them equally to lower urinary tract symptoms, the higher incidence of bladder outlet obstruction in men as a result of prostatic enlargement has significant influence on the worsened voiding symptoms in men. But enlargement of the prostate is not the only problem, it is the combination of alterations of detrusor function and obstruction. In 160 men with lower urinary tract symptoms, pure bladder outlet obstruction was found in 55% whereas 45% of these men had outlet obstruction and an overactive bladder (Knutson et al. 2001). This correlates with urodynamic investigations by Collas et Malone-Lee reporting significant reduction in bladder compliance and maximal capacity asso-ciated with an increase in bladder capacity at first desire to void in females between 20–90 years (Collas and Malone-Lee 1996). Alterations in bladder storage and emptying function cause urgency and frequency and may finally lead to incontinence. These changes have significant impact on the quality of life associated with the feeling of physical infirmity, depression, and isolation. In a recent rural Japanese study of more than 2000 people older than 65 years the rate of urinary incontinence in homebound elderly men and women was 4.7% and 11.3%. These results are comparable to others (Daha et al. 2002, Yarnell and StLeger 1979). The rate of incontinence in nursing home residents increased from 16.2% to 23.2%. Incontinence was predominately urge related in 66% of men and more than 50% in women. Although men often complained of voiding symptoms, incontinence did not have major impact on daily activities in this Japanese cohort. In contrast, women hesitated to participate in group excursions and outdoor exercise, and had a tendency to live alone or indoors. But one very important finding was that 81.5% of "patients" complaining of incontinence did not visit a doctor. This again supports the hypothesis that aging is associated with an increased acceptance of infirmities, considering them as a natural process. According to Madersbacher et al., only 5% of women and 16% of men looked for treatment after complaining of incontinence for more than three years (Madersbacher 2000). This is consistent with others showing that only 66% of incontinent men and women seek therapy, 1/3 accept it as an aging infirmity (Barlow et al. 1997, Milsom et al. 2001).

Although aging people are often bothered by their voiding symptoms, some will not look for relief. One reason that older women often do not talk about their incontinence is embarrassment or the belief that there is no cure (Butler et al. 1999). Therefore, it is the doctor who should ask about voiding symptoms including loss of urine that may not be cured in all cases but can usually be improved. In a large survey on more than 6000 German patients older than 50 years, patients were interviewed if their doctors asked them about urinary incontinence (Welz-Barth et al. 2000). It was found that doctors were less likely to address this issue in 1999 compared with 1996, thus withholding appropriate care from incontinent patients. It was hypothesized that possible reasons for these were financial restrictions of health budgets and/or a lack of appreciation of problems associated with incontinence among doctors and/or health policy makers. But not only the doctors are responsible for this dilemma since 25% of incontinent patients older than 50 years still keep it secret from their doctor (Welz-Barth et al. 2000).

Besides medical treatment of incontinence, additional incontinence device are often required. Kirshen estimated in 1983 that 20% of the aging population in Canada has urinary incontinence causing a minimum of $150 million for incontinence pads (Kirshen 1983). In the United States, the annual direct costs of urinary incontinence was estimated as $16.3 billion, with 76% of these costs required for incontinence in women and 24% for men (Wilson et al. 2001). In Sweden, estimated annual costs for incontinence devices accounts for 0.5% of total costs of Swedish healthcare and 0,05% of the gross national product (Samuelsson 2001). Consistent with the fact that 90% of healthcare expenditure is incurred in the last 10 years of life, the costs for incontinence in women over 65 years were more than twice the costs of women under 65 in the US (Wilson et al. 2001). The largest cost category was routine care (70%), followed by nursing home admissions (14%), treatment (9%), complications (6%), and diagnosis and evaluations (1%) (Wilson et al. 2001). Considering that urgency and frequency are the most distressing symptom of the aging bladder detrusor in both men and women, Stewart et al. reported on total costs estimated at $12.6 billion in 2000 for the treatment of overactive bladder (Stewart et al. 2002). These enormous expenses emphasise the importance for the treatment of the aging detrusor to relieve patients symptoms, improve quality of life, probably reduce depression, and reduce healthcare costs.

3.   Urinary tract infections

In addition to an increase in frequency, urgency, nocturia, bladder outlet obstruction, vaginal itching, and urogenital atrophy during aging, infections of the lower genitourinary tract are seen more commonly in elderly men and women. Prevalence of urinary tract infections differ between men and women throughout lifetime with a higher frequency in women than men. However, during aging, infection rates become comparable, equalising in the population over the age of 65 years (Boscia et al. 1986, Lipsky 1989). In a survey on more than 7309 consultations in our outpatient clinic between 1996 and 1997, patients older than 80 years suffered 36.5% from urinary tract infections (Daha et al. 2002). Pathogenesis of these infections are multifactorial such as bladder outlet obstruction, prostate enlargement, residual urine, decreased antibacterial activity of prostatic secretion, indwelling catheters, urothelial- and vaginal atrophy (Boscia et al. 1986, Lipsky 1989). This may be related to the menopause and its duration in aging women. Besides these components, general immunodeficiency has been suggested in elderly patients (Stamey 1980, Gardner 1980).

4.   Tumours, cancer, and aging

Bladder outlet obstruction concomitant with prostate enlargement is a well known phenomenon in aging men affecting nearly every man older than 80 years. Men > 80 years have a prevalence of benign prostatic hyperplasia of 75–90% (Moore 1944, Walsh 1992). This process is thought to start at about 50 years of age, with 26.9% of men reporting moderate lower urinary tract symptoms and only 2.8% suffering from severe symptoms (Madersbacher et al. 1998). As expected, bladder outlet obstruction and symptoms correlate well with age since surgical interventions increased in aging men (Glynn et al. 1985). However, 33% of men in their 60s and 70s accept their voiding symptoms and do not seek special medical care (Ekman 1989).

Aging is associated not only with benign diseases of the genitourinary tract but also with a significant increase in cancer ratios compared with younger ages. Men and women older than 65 years have the greatest burden of cancer since 55% of all malignancies develop in this age group (Yanik and Ries 1994). The incidence in elderly patients has been reported as 2085 per 100 000 compared with 194 per 100 000 in patients younger than 65 (Yanik and Ries 1991). But risk numbers significantly increase with aging since people older than 65 are at a 10 times greater risk to develop cancer as individuals younger than 65 years.

Cancers of the lower genitourinary tract are seen often (Vercelli et al. 1999). With regard to cancer specific sites in men, the bladder and prostate had the highest prevalence five years from diagnosis (more than 800 cases per 100 000) followed by colon, lung (about 500 cases per 100 000), stomach, and rectum (about 300 cases per 100 000) (Vercelli et al. 1999). Prostate cancer is the second major cause of death in men in most countries, but it is already the major cause of death in men over the age of 50 in other countries, with a prevalence of 15%. With cancer progression, lower urinary tract symptoms may emerge, such as outlet obstruction and urgency. Although the incidence of prostate cancer increases with age, a decreased death rate has been reported in geriatric patients compared with younger men (Chodak et al. 1994). In women, breast cancer ranked first (more than 1,000 cases per 100 000) followed by colon (about 350 cases per 100 000), corpus uteri, stomach, and rectum cancers (between 150 and 200 cases per 100 000) (Vercelli et al. 1999). These figures confirm the important role of aging in cancer development.

Since tumours and cancers of the lower genitourinary tract have a significant impact on voiding symptoms, new strategies will be necessary to improve therapies and again may relieve at least in part lower urinary tract symptoms.

5.   Closing remarks

Symptoms of the lower genitourinary tract are frequently seen in aging men and women. Irrespective of differences in sex, most distressing are urinary frequency, urgency, and nocturia, followed by dysuria, vaginal itching, and local burning sensations. The prevalence of urinary tract infections differs between men and women throughout lifetime with a higher frequency in women than men. But with aging infection rates become comparable between both sexes, evening out in the population over the age of 65 years. Although there is a high prevalence of symptoms, 33% of symptomatic patients do not seek therapy, either because of acceptance of their infirmity as normal age-related process, misinformation, or sometimes a lack of interest on the part of the physician. In order to treat and probably prevent distressing voiding dysfunctions of the aging bladder detrusor, new strategies and investigations will be necessary to improve therapeutic options. This is of utmost importance to the often affected aging population but also for healthcare budgets since incontinence incurs significant expense.

Changes of the aging bladder are commonly seen in daily practice that can be treated. New aspects and therapeutic options may increase opportunities to diminish symptoms from the aging bladder to improve quality of life and decrease costs for incontinence devices. Investigations should focus on quality of life improvement to enable healthy aging of for men and women.

6.   References

1. Badelt C, Holzmann-Jenkins A, Matul C, Österle A (1996) Kosten der Pflegesicherung. Strukturen und Entwicklungstrends der Altenbetreuung, 2. Aufl. Böhlau: Wien
2. Barlow DH, Samsioe G, van Geelen JM (1997) A study of European womens' experience of the problems of urogenital aging and its management. Maturitas 27: 239–247

3. Boscia JA, Kobasa WD, Knight RA, Abrutyn E, Levison ME, Kaye D (1986) Epidemiology of bacteriuria in an elderly ambulatory population. Am J Med 80: 208–214
4. Busby-Whitehead JM, Johnson TM (1998) Urinary incontinence. Clin Geriatr Med 14: 285–296
5. Butler RN, Maby JI, Montella JM, Young GP (1999) Urinary incontinence: keys to diagnosis of the older woman. Geriatrics 54: 22–26
6. Campbell AJ, Reinken J, McCosh L (1985) Incontinence in the elderly: prevalence and prognosis. Age Aging 14: 65–70
7. Carbone A, Gezeroglu H, Aloisi P, Mander A, Osborn J (2001) Is aging real risk factor for urological pathologies in men and women? Arch Esp Urol 54: 87–94
8. Chodak GW, Thisted RA, Gerbber GS, Johansson JE, Adolfsson J, Jones GW, Chisholm GD, Moskovitz B, Livne PM, Warner J (1994) Results of conservative management of clinically localized prostate cancer. N Engl J Med 330: 242–248
9. Collas DM, Malone-Lee JG (1996) Age-associated changes in detrusor sensory function in women with lower urinary tract symptoms. Int Urogynecol J Pelvic Floor Dysfunct 7: 24–29
10. Daha LK, Riedl CR, Simak R, Engelhardt PF, Plas E, Pflüger H (2002) Incidence of urologic diseases in geriatric patients in a large community hospital. J Am Geriatr Soc (in press)
11. Ekman P (1989) BPH epidemiology and risk factors. Prostate [Suppl] 2: 23–31
12. Gardner ID (1980) The effect of aging on susceptibility to infection. Rev Infect Dis 2: 801–810
13. Glynn RJ, Campion EW, Bouchard GR, Silbert JE (1985) The development of benign prostatic hyperplasia among volunteers in the normative aging study. Am J Epidemiol 121: 78–90
14. Hampel C, Wienhold D, Benken N, Eggersmann C, Thüroff JW (1997) Definition of overactive bladder and epidemiology of urinary incontinence. Urology 50 [Suppl] 6A: 4–14
15. Kakizaki H, Matsuura S, Mitsui T, Ameda K, Tanaka H, Koyanagi T (2002) Questionnaire analysis on sex difference in lower urinary tract symptoms. Urology 59: 58–62
16. Kirshen AJ (1983) Urinary incontinence in the elderly: a review. Clin Invest Med 6: 331–339
17. Knutson T, Edlund C, Fall M, Dahlstrand C (2001) BPH with coexisting overactive bladder dysfunction – an everyday urological dilemma. Neurourol Urodyn 20: 237–247
18. Koyama W, Koyanagi A, Mihara S, Kawazu S, Uemura T, Nakano H, Gotou Y, Nishizawa M, Noyama A, Hasegawa C, Nakano M (1998) Prevalence and conditions of urinary incontinence among the elderly. Methods Inf Med 37: 151–155
19. Langa KM, Fultz NH, Saint S, Kabeto MU, Herzog AR (2002) Informal caregiving time and costs for urinary incontinence in older individuals in the United States. J Am Geriatr Soc 50: 733–737
20. Lipsky BA (1989) Urinary tract infections in men: Epidemiology, pathophysiology, diagnosis, and treatment. Ann Intern Med 110: 138–150
21. Madersbacher S (2000) Prevalence of lower urinary tract symptoms and urinary incontinence in the elderly: recent data from Austria. Wien Klin Wochenschr 112: 379–380

22. Madersbacher S, Haidinger G, Temml C, Schmidbauer CP (1998) Prevalence of lower urinary tract symptoms in Austria as assessed by an open survey of 2,096 men. Eur Urol 34: 136–141
23. Milsom I, Abrams P, Cardozo L, Roberts RG, Thüroff JW, Wein AJ (2001) How widespread are the symptoms of an overactive bladder and how are they managed? A population-based prevalence study. BJU Int 87: 760–766
24. Moore RA (1944) Benign hypertrophy and carcinoma of the prostate. Surgery 16: 152–676
25. Olshansky SJ, Carnes BA, Cassel CK (1991) In search of Methuselah: Estimating the upper limits to human longevity. Science 250: 634–640
26. Resnick NM (1987) Urinary incontinence. Public Health Rep [Suppl]: 67–70
27. Romanzi LJ (2001) Urinary incontinence in women and men. J Gend Specif Med 4: 14–20
28. Samuelsson E, Mansson L, Milsom I (2001) Incontinence aids in Sweden: users and costs. BJU Int 88: 893–898
29. Schmeiser-Rieder A, Kunze M (1999) Viennese Men's Health Report 1999
30. Stamey TA (1980) Pathogenesis and treatment of urinary tract infections. Williams & Wilkins: Baltimore
31. Stewart K, McGhan WF, Offerdahl T, Corey R (2002) Overactive bladder patients and role of the pharmacist. J Am Pharm Assoc 42: 469–476
32. Tseng IJ, Chen YT, Chen MT, Kou HY, Tseng SF (2000) Prevalence of urinary incontinence and intention to seek treatment in the elderly. J Formos Med Assoc 99: 753–758
33. Vercelli M, Quaglia A, Parodi S, Crosignani P (1999) Cancer prevalence in the elderly. ITAPREVAL Working Group. Tumori 85: 391–399
34. Walsh PC (1992) Benign prostatic hyperplasia. In: Walsh PC, Retik AB, Stamey TA, et al (eds) Campbell's urology, 6 edn. WB Saunders: Philadelphia, pp 1009
35. Welz-Barth A, Füsgen I, Melchior HJ (2000) 1999 rerun of the 1996 German urinary incontinence in the elderly. World J Urol 18: 436–438
36. Wilson L, Brown JS, Shin GP, Luc KO, Subak LL (2001) Annual direct cost of urinary incontinence. Obstet Gynecol 98: 398–406
37. World Health Organization Aging and Life Course (2001) Men, Aging and Health
38. Yanik R, Ries LG (1991) Cancer in the aged. An epidemiologic perspective on treatment issues. Cancer 68 [Suppl] 11: 2502–2510
39. Yanik R, Ries LA (1994) Cancer in older persons. Magnitude of the problem – how do we apply what we know? Cancer 74 [Suppl] 7: 1995–2003
40. Yarnell JWG, StLeger AS (1979) The prevalence, severity and factors associated with urinary incontinence in a random sample of the elderly. Age Aging 8: 81–85

Correspondence address: Lukas K Daha, MD, Department of Urology and LBI for Urology & Andrology, Lainz Hospital, Vienna, Wolkersbergenstrasse 1, A-1130 Vienna (E-mail: kurosch.daha@wienkav.at).

Morphology and ultrastructure of the aging bladder

M. Susani

Department of Clinical Pathology, University of Vienna, General Hospital of Vienna, Vienna, Austria

Contents

1.   Introduction

The functional inconvenience of aging bladder is outlet obstruction, reduced bladder capacity and incontinence. Normal urinary bladder function depends on adequate extensibility during the filling phase without involuntary contractions of the smooth muscles by simultaneously keeping the sphincter closed. For voiding an adequate force of muscle constriction is necessary by simultaneously opening the bladder outlet. This function depends mainly on the smooth muscles of the bladder wall – also called detrusor – and its neural supply and control. Therefore the muscle cells need an adequate force of contraction, a complex architecture arranged in fascicles, and a normal innervation. Impaired bladder function is either caused by detrusor dysfunction or results from the effect of neurogenic disorders or obstruction. Functional pathology of the urinary bladder therefore focuses on the light and electron microscopic changes of the detrusor. According to the work of Ahmed Elbadawi there is a concept to interpretate these findings and to get relevant information on the kind of voiding dysfunction. The cited literature at the end of this article is restricted mainly to this author because his investigations have a practical diagnostic approach. In a pilot study at our place this concept turned out to be highly useful and reproducible even by pathologists not yet experienced in this diagnostic field.

The method of the diagnostic procedure is described. The morphological findings in the normal urinary bladder are compared to changes in the detrusor of patients with voiding disorders. The characteristics of four different groups defined by electron microscopic changes and their functional correlates are summarised.

2. Normal histology of the urinary bladder detrusor

2.1 Light microscopy

The detrusor of the urinary bladder body, also called muscularis propria, consists of three integrative tissue compartments, smooth muscle, interstitium containing blood vessels, collagen fibrils, elastic fibrils, basement membrane material, and intrinsic nerves. The muscle cells are arranged in compact bundles. The orientation of the muscle cells is the same in each bundle. Bundles are organised in fascicles, which were incompletely separated by microseptae (Fig. 1A).

2.2 Ultrastructure

The detrusor has the ultrastructural features of smooth muscle cells with cylindrical configuration. The contour is smooth in relaxed cells. The sarcolemma (cell membrane) is alternatively thick and thin. The thick zones (dense bands) consist of sarcolemma with adjacent electron dense material to which myofilaments are attached. These areas are of functional importance to transmit the contraction force to the interstitium and the surrounding cells. The thin zones consist of sarcolemma with strings of caveolae, appearing as flask shaped surface vesicles of uniform size (Fig. 1D). In this areas the active ion transport and the exchange of Na^+/Ca^{++} takes place, which is necessary for excitation and the following contraction. The sarcoplasma contains myofilaments with evenly dispersed dense bodies.

Within the fascicles the muscle cells are separated by a space of uniform width usually less than 200 NM. In the intercellular space basal lamina material, isolated collagen fibrils and rare elastic fibrils are found. The contact between muscle cells is formed by intermediate junctions (zonulae adherentes), built up of parallel opposed sarcolemmae of two neighbouring cells with a separating gap 40–70 NM wide (Fig. 1C). Desmosomes and gap junctions are usually absent in the normal detrusor.

Schwann cell ensheathed axons extend along the microseptae. Neuroeffector junctions with muscle cells are established by bare axons, which are packed with synaptic vesicles. They appear clear in cholinergic and electron dense in adrenergic nerves. The distance between axon and sarcolemma in this kind of junction is 15–80 NM (Fig. 1B).

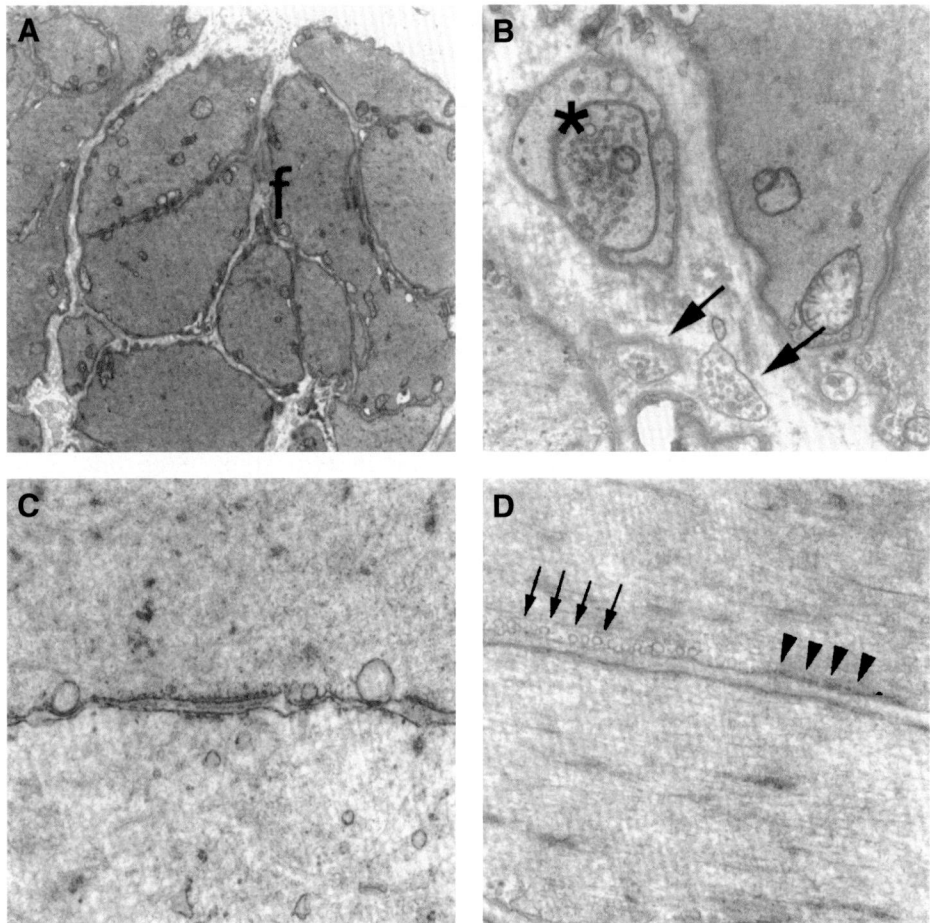

Fig. 1. A The normal detrusor is arranged in muscle cell bundles, which are organized in fascicles. Arrows – microseptae, *f* fascicle. **B** Inervation of the detrusor: Schwann cell ensheathed axon situated in a microsepta (asterisk). Bare axons (arrows) containing clear cholinergic vesicles forming up a neuroeffector junction with a muscle cell. **C** Intermediate junction between two muscles cells. **D** Sarcolemma of a normal muscle cell with alternating thick zones (thick arrows) built up by attached myofilaments and thin zones with are rich in caveolae (thin arrows)

3. Clinico-pathological presumption for a morphological analysis of voiding disorders

Specific and different ultrastructural changes in one or more tissue compartments of the detrusor mirror an abnormal detrusor function. These ultrastructure patterns are additive when different abnormalities coexist. This presumption was proven to be valid by Elbadawi and make it possible to diagnose different voiding dysfunctions on endoscopic detrusor biopsies.

The important technical presumptions are carefully taken biopsies and well preserved and accurately fixed tissue. One method for the biopsy procedure is endoscopic cold cup biopsy, taken from a short distance above and lateral to one ureteric orifice. The second is a percutaneous, trans-abdominal, ultrasound guided, detrusor biopsy from the anterior wall of the full bladder. An automatic biopsy device using a 14G needle of 22 mm length is recommended (Holm 1996). The tissue has to be fixed immediately in 2.5% glutaraldehyde in cacodylate buffer. The buffer solution has to be free of Ca^{++} ions to avoid muscular contractions. Such contractions result in ultrastructural muscle cell profiles with crenellated contours that would hinder the evaluation of important parameters and structural details. The muscle cells should be sectioned longitudinally or oblique to their long axis. Such sections are suited best for evaluation of cell junctions, caveolae, and dense bands of sarcolemma and the content of intercellular space.

Histological evaluation has to be done in two steps. Step one is to determine the uniform or focally different architecture of the detrusor and the structural type of its muscle fascicles. Three types of muscle fascicles can be observed, which are discerned on the degree of separation of the individual muscle cells, the content of spaces separating the muscle cells, and the kind of muscle cell junctions. The normal *compact fascicle* profile has closely arranged muscle cells, frequent and easily found intermediate cell junctions and a narrow empty- appearing intercellular compartment. This contains basal lamina-like material and loosely arranged individual collagen fibrils, but no collagenous or elastic fibres. The *intermediate fascicle* shows mildly and unevenly separated muscle cells. The intercellular space contains more basal lamina material, more collagen fibrils and rare elastic microfibrils, but still no elastic fibres. Intermediate junctions are recognized sporadically. Protrusion cell junctions and ultraclose abutments may be frequent. Moderate to marked muscle cell separation with wide intercellular space containing abundant aggregated collagen fibrils and occasional fibers characterizes the *loose fascicle*. Aggregates of elastic microfibrils are common few or many elastic fibres may be seen. Protrusion cell junctions and ultraclose abutments are usually frequent. Step two identifies ultra-structural changes on the cellular level specific for an overactive, obstructed or a detrusor with impaired contractility or simply patterns of aging.

4. Changes of the aging urinary bladder without severe functional consequence

The *dense-band pattern* was identified as the distinctive ultrastructure of the old urinary bladder (Elbadavi et al. 1993b). The changes were found in a group of 65–96 years old patients. They were continent asymptomatic, urodynami-cally stable; the bladder was normally contractile and unobstructed.

Muscle cell fascicles have a normal arrangement and a compact structure; the spaces between the muscle cells are slightly widened, with a limited content of collagen fibrils. The configuration of the muscle cells is

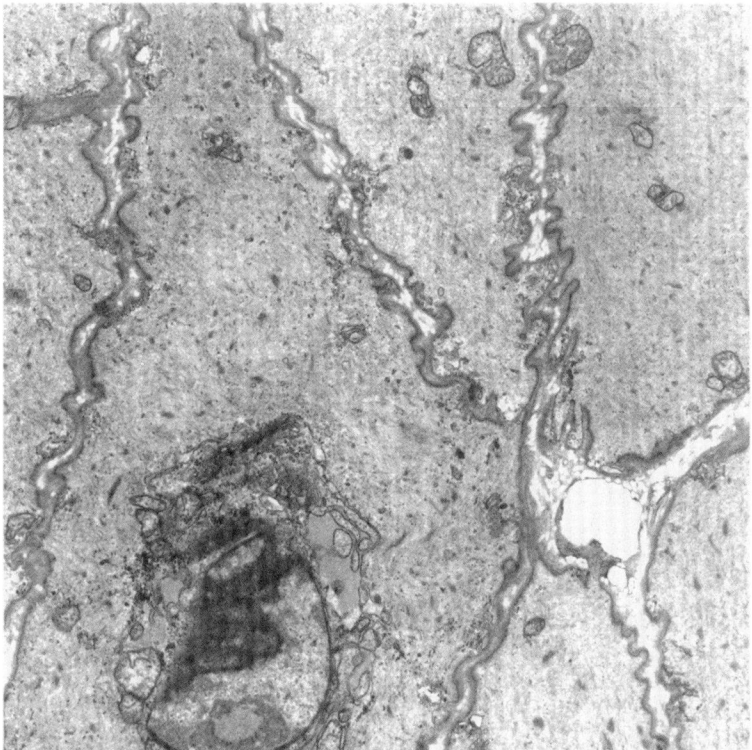

Fig. 2. Detrusor with normally arranged muscle cells. Long dense bands dominate their sarcolemma

cylindrical and their contours are smooth. The individual cells are in contact by intermediate junctions. But muscle cell membranes are dominated by very long dense bands, whereas the thin areas with caveolae are markedly depleted (Fig. 2).

This depletion of caveolae in the aged detrusor may indicate a process of degeneration. Differentiation of smooth muscle cells is associated with progressively increasing numbers of caveolae. Dedifferentiation reverts mature cells from an active contractile to an inactive synthetic phenotype of immature cells. This reversion is associated with reduction of caveolae, reduction of myofilaments, expansion of endoplasmatic reticulum and increased synthesis and secretion of extra cellular matrix proteins as collagen and elastin (Campell GR 1990). It could be expected that depletion of caveolae in the dense band pattern detrusor results in changes of contractility, but these changes might be too subtle to be detected urodynamically.

5.   Detrusor weakness – degenerative pattern

Wide spread degenerative changes in all components of the detrusor as smooth muscle cells, and axons are the morphological equivalent for impaired contractility. Two grades of severity could be discerned, a *disruptive* and a *non-disruptive degenerative pattern* judged on the condition and continuity of intracytoplasmatic myofilaments. Limited forms of degeneration patterns are confined to single cells or small cell groups and may be seen in combination with the dense band pattern of the aging bladder without severe functional consequences.

The fascicular organization of the muscle cells is preserved and the interstitium is not altered very much. The intercellular space is variably widened, but the cells often retain their intermediate junctions with intact or degenerated cells. Axons and axon terminals are also degenerated with depletion of synaptic vesicles. The axoplasma is cleared, and may contain multivesicular bodies or dens patches. Some axolemmas are disrupted. Ultimately axon lysis or fragmentation occurs.

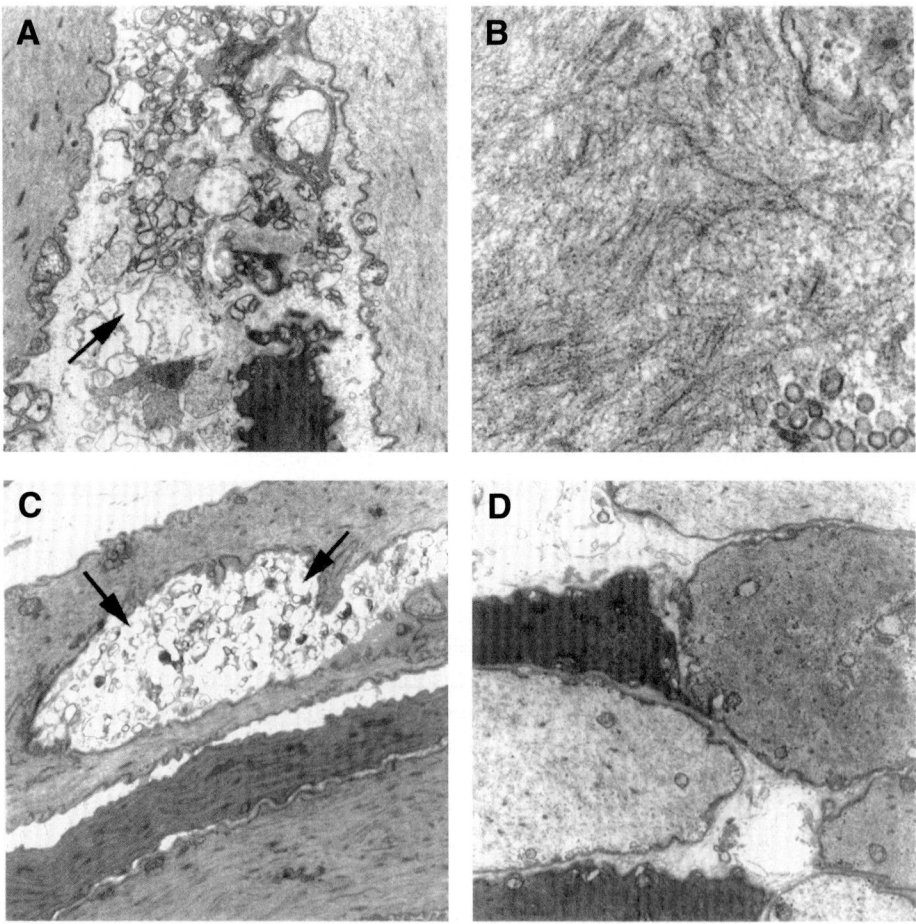

Fig. 3. Degenerative pattern. **A** Degenerated smooth muscle cell (arrow). **B** Irregularly criss cross-arranged myofilaments. **C** Vacuolated Smooth muscle cell (arrow). **D** Mosaic pattern of very dark and pale smooth muscle cells

Disorganization and disruption of myofilaments define "disruptive degeneration pattern". Other intracytoplasmatic phenomena of degeneration as sarcoplasmatic dense bodies, disrupted mitochondria, microcystic distention of endoplasmatic reticulum and lamellar bodies are present. In more severe degeneration muscle cells become intensively dark or lysed (Fig. 3A, D) and fragmented.

A less severe form is the non-disruptive *degeneration pattern*, which shows more subtle alterations. Myofilaments exhibit misalignment with disarray, patchy stacking, crisscrossing and swerving (Fig. 3B). Sarcoplasmic dense bodies are often crowded and clumped.

6.   Hyperactive detrusor – dysjunctional pattern

Complete dysjunctional pattern is the morphological correlate for an overactive detrusor, which is characterised by involuntary spontaneous contractions of a limited number of muscle cells. The *incomplete dysjunctional pattern* is confined to single smooth muscle cells with abnormal cell junctions in the minority, most junctions were of normal intermediate type. This quantitatively less severe form has usually no functional consequence.

The muscle fascicles are readily discernable and are usually of intermediate type. They are varying a little in size and in the compactness of arrangement. The muscle cells are slightly unevenly separated, with a higher amount of collagen fibres or fibrils and only a slight increase of elastic material.

On the cellular level there is a marked reduction or loss of normal intermediate muscle junctions. Unique protrusion junctions and simple ultraclose abutments mediate the contact between muscle cells. The cytoplasm of individual muscle cells are protruded and form long slender finger like or piliform processes extending from one muscle cell towards a neighbouring cell (Fig. 4A). The contact zones form very narrow gaps of 9 NM or less appearing as pseudosyncytium in low magnification. 5–12 muscle cells connected in this kind form chains (Fig. 4B). In the normal contractile overactive detrusor the intrinsic nerves and neuroeffector junctions are normal.

Depletion of normal cell junctions impede the mechanical coupling of detrusor muscle cells, the mechanism that normally transmits the contraction force from one cell to the next. The narrow gap junctions like cell connections enable groups of cells for very fast electric coupling leading to spontaneously, stretch evoked or neural triggered contraction of isolated muscle cell groups.

7.   Outlet obstruction – obstructive pattern

Obstruction results in the '*myohypertrophy pattern*', which is characteristically patchy in extent and degree. In combination with extreme impairment of contractility it results in overdistention.

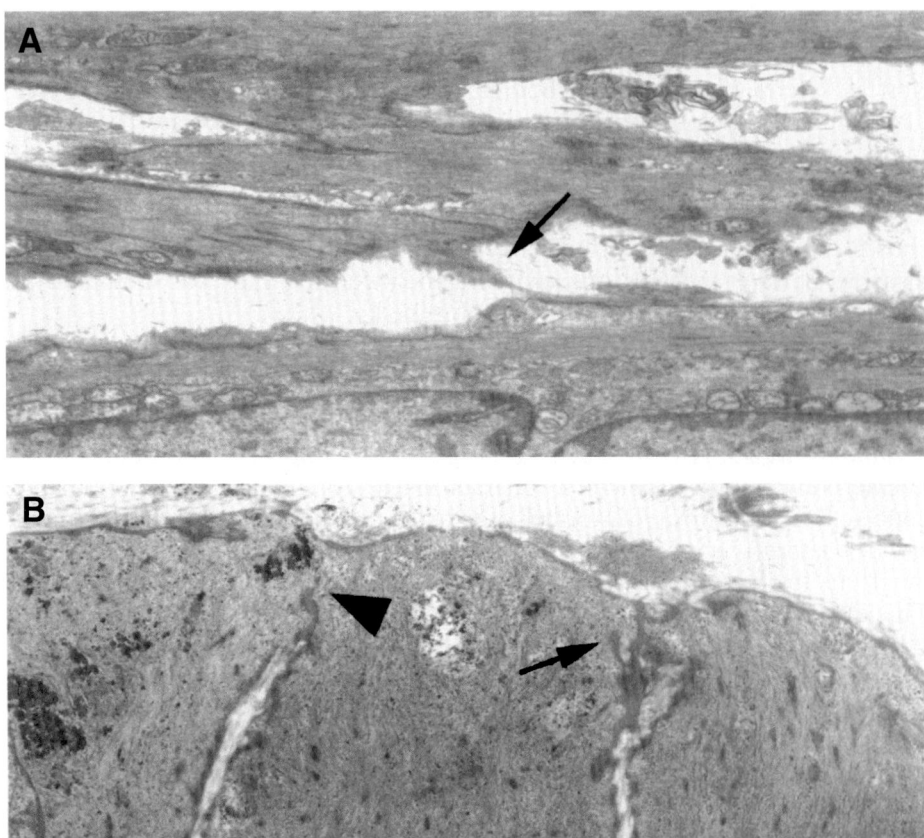

Fig. 4. **A** Finger like projection forming a narrow contact with the neighbouring cell (arrow) characteristic for a dysjunctional pattern. **B** A chain of three smooth muscle cells with very narrow contact zones (arrow) and a syncytium like connection on the left (arrowhead)

The muscle cell arrangement is severely disturbed and gets the characteristics of a loose fascicle. The individual cells are widely separated; intermediate junctions are hard to find. The wide intercellular spaces contain collagen fibrils and fibres as well as elastic fibres. These fibres are associated with fibroblasts containing an expended endoplasmatic reticulum and abundant mitochondria. Chronic overdistention develops a characteristic "hyperelastosis pattern". In this subset of myohypertrophy shows an extreme widening of the intercellular space, containing a big amount of collagen and prominent elastic fibres. The fascicular arrangement of muscle cells is vaguely discernable or lost.

Hypertrophic muscle cells are big, their profiles are bizarre, branched, and braided. Hypertrophy can be suspected without morphometry with a

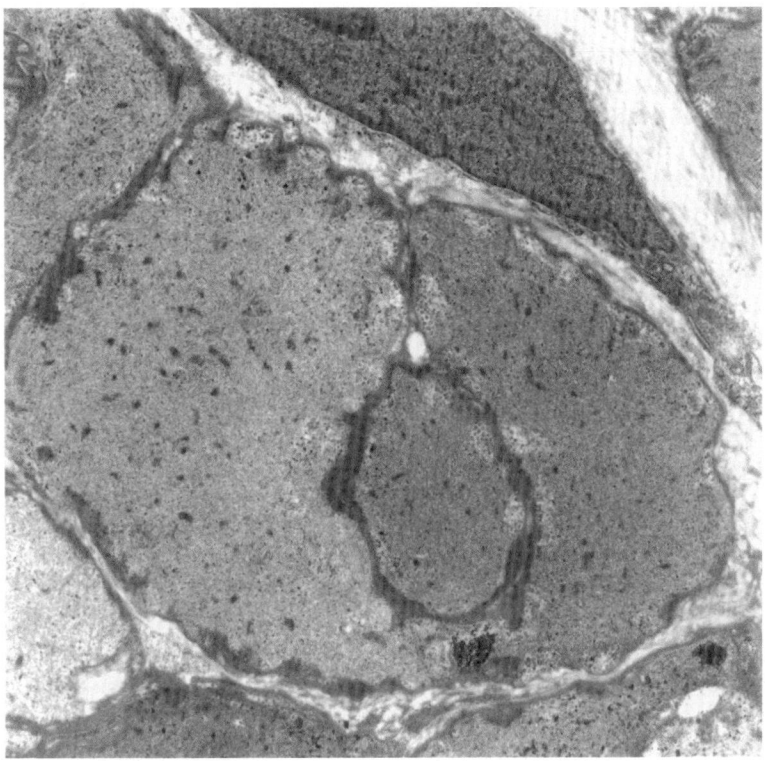

Fig. 5. Hypertrophic muscle cell wrapped over another as a typical finding in the obstructive pattern

high level of certainty, when extreme variability in profile diameters exceeding the range of 3 times the smallest is observed in the same microscopic field. Bizarre cells have convoluted contour and are wrapped around one or more other cell profiles (Fig. 5) or may be contorted. Cell branching and braiding can be seen only in longitudinally or oblique sectioned profiles. Different orientation of myofilaments within the muscle cells of one fascicle is a characteristic feature of hypertrophy.

The detrusor initially adjusting to the bladder outlet obstruction develops severe alterations. These changes in the following act as active contributor to the voiding dysfunction and result in the ultimate destruction of the bladder function.

8. Closing remarks

Functional pathology of the detrusor is a challenge for two main reasons. One reason is the medical importance related to demographic aspects of worldwide population development. Elderly people can suffer from severe voiding dysfunction, which may lead to social isolation. Therefore treatment and diagnosis are of major interest. The other reason is that ultrastructural analysis of detrusor biopsies enables diagnosis on the kind of functional disturbance such as detrusor hyperactivity, obstruction, or degeneration. This is rather unique, because morphology is an excellent tool for discerning different kinds of pathological processes or tumours but not to get insight functional activity of organ systems.

Ultrastructural analysis can differentiate myogenic alterations of the detrusor associated with aging, haveing no functional consequences from degenerative processes combined with detrusor weakness, hyperactivity with the dysjunctional pattern, and the hypertrophic pattern of outlet obstruction. This method requires a well functioning electron microscopic laboratory, which is not available for most doctors treating the patients. This may be one reason that this method is not widely used. So far, it is unclear if morphological analysis of the detrusor in addition to urodynamic investigations will add new information for drawing specific therapeutic conclusions.

9. References

1. Campell GR, Campell JH (1990) Ultrasrtucture of smooth muscle cells in culture. In: Motta PM (ed) Ultrastructure of smooth muscle. Kluwer, Boston, pp 79–99
2. Elbadavi A (1993) Functional pathology of urinary bladder muscularis: the new frontier in diagnostic uropathology. Sem Diag Path 10: 314–354
3. Elbadavi A, Diokono AC, Millard RJ (1998) The aging bladder: Morphology and urodynamics. World J Urol 16: S10–S34
4. Elbadavi A, Heilemariam S, Yalla SV, Resnick NM (1997) Structural basis of geriatric voiding dysfunction. VI. Validation and update of diagnostic criteria in 71 detrusor biopsies. J Urol 157: 1802–1813
5. Elbadavi A, Heilemariam S, Yalla SV, Resnick NM (1997) Structural basis of geriatric voiding dysfunction. VII. Prospective ultrastructural/urodynamic evaluation of its natural evolution. J Urol 157: 1814–1822
6. Elbadavi A, Yalla SV, Resnick NM (1993) Structural basis of geriatric voiding dysfunction. II. Aging detrusor: normal vs. impaired contractility. J Urol 150: 1657–1667
7. Heilemariam S, Elbadawi A, Yalla SV, Resnick NM (1997) Structural basis of geriatric voiding dysfunction. V. Standardized protocols for routine ultrastructural study and diagnosis of endoscopic detrusor biopsies. J Urol 157: 1783–1801
8. Holm NR, Horn T, Elbadavi A, Skjoldby B, Nordling J (1996) A new technique for detrusor biopsy and its applicability in the ultrastructural study and diagnosis of voiding dysfunction. Brit J Urol 77: 785–791

Correspondence address: Martin Susani, MD, Department of Clinical Pathology, University of Vienna, General Hospital of Vienna, Währinger Gürtel 18–20, A-1090 Vienna, Austria (E-mail: martin.susani@akh-wien.ac.at).

Muscarinic receptors and the aging bladder

K.-E. Andersson

Department of Clinical Pharmacology, Lund University Hospital, Lund, Sweden

Contents

1.   Introduction

The prevalence of the overactive bladder (OAB) syndrome, characterised by symptoms of urgency, with and without urge incontinence, usually with frequency and nocturia (Abrams et al. 2002), increases with age (Milsom et al. 2001). In western Europe, OAB was estimated to occur in nearly 17% of the population (Milsom et al. 2001), and detrusor overactivity is often the underlying condition. The three most common pathophysiological mechanisms in geriatric voiding dysfunction are obstruction, detrusor instability, and impaired detrusor contraction (Hald and Horn 1998). Muscarinic receptors are involved in both normal and disturbed bladder contraction, and the most common drug treatment of OAB is antimuscarinic drugs (Andersson et al. 2002). Age related changes in muscarinic receptor functions and in the bladder activation mechanisms may therefore be of particular therapeutic interest. However, the details of both the muscarinic receptor functions and the bladder activation mechanisms, normally and in different age related bladder disorders, remain to be established (de Groat and Yoshimura 2001, Andersson 2002). Below, normal bladder activation is briefly discussed, as are changes in muscarinic receptors related to age and to disorders common in elderly people and associated with OAB.

2. Muscarinic receptor mechanisms

2.1 Muscarinic receptors

Muscarinic receptors comprise five subtypes, encoded by five distinct genes (Caulfield and Birdsall 1998). The five gene products correspond to pharmacologically defined receptors, and M_1–M_5 is used to describe both the molecular and pharmacological subtypes. Muscarinic receptors are coupled to G-proteins, but the signal transduction systems vary (Caulfield and Birdsall 1998). M_1, M_3, and M_5 receptors couple preferentially to $G_{q/11}$, activating phosphoinositide hydrolysis, in turn leading to mobilisation of intracellular calcium. M_2 and M_4 receptors couple to pertussis toxin-sensitive $G_{i/o}$, resulting in inhibition of adenylyl cyclase activity. M_2 receptor stimulation may also activate non-specific cation channels (Kotlikoff et al. 1999) and inhibit K_{ATP} channels through activation of protein kinase C (Bonev and Nelson 1993).

2.2 Muscarinic receptors and normal bladder contraction

Normal human bladder contraction is mediated mainly through stimulation of muscarinic receptors in the detrusor muscle (Andersson 1993, Yamanishi et al. 2001). The human detrusor contains muscarinic receptors of the M_2 and M_3 subtype (Hegde and Eglen 1999, Eglen et al. 2001), with M_2 receptors (2/3) dominating quantitatively over M_3 receptors (1/3). However, the M_3 receptors are responsible mainly for the normal micturition contraction (Hegde and Eglen 1999, Eglen et al. 2001, Yamanishi et al. 2002). In mice lacking the M_3 receptor, carbachol induced contractions were mediated by M_2 receptors (Matsui et al. 2000). However, the contractile amplitude of the carbachol induced contractions of isolated detrusor strips was only 5% of that found in normal bladders.

The role for the M_2 receptors in bladder function has not been established. It has been suggested that M_2 receptors may oppose sympathetically (via β-adrenoceptors) mediated relaxation of the smooth muscle, since activation of M_2 receptors results in an inhibition of adenylyl cyclase (Hegde et al. 1997, Yamanishi et al. 2002). As mentioned previously, stimulation of M_2 receptors may, in addition, activate non-specific cationic channels and inactivate potassium channels.

Muscarinic receptors can be found on the pre-synaptic nerve terminals and participate in the regulation of transmitter release, and may be both inhibitory and excitatory. The inhibitory pre-junctional receptor has been classified as M_2 in animal (Somogyi and de Groat 1992, Tobin and Sjögren 1998), and as M_4 in the human bladder (D'Agostino et al. 2000). The facilitatory muscarinic receptor seems to be of the M_1 subtype in animal, and probably also in human, bladders (Somogyi and de Groat 1992, 1999; Tobin and Sjögren 1998).

2.3   Muscarinic receptors and age-related bladder dysfunction

2.3.1   Outflow obstruction

Outflow obstruction is common in elderly men and may change the cholinergic functions of the bladder. Reduced cholinergic innervation of the obstructed bladder wall has been shown in several species, including humans (Gosling et al. 1986, Sibley 1987, Speakman et al. 1987, Pandita et al. 2000). In pigs with experimental outflow obstruction, the detrusor response to intramural nerve stimulation was decreased. However, a supersensitivity of the detrusor to acetylcholine (ACh) could be demonstrated (Sibley 1987). In detrusor muscle of obstructed patients with bladder instability, similar changes were found (Harrison et al. 1987). It was suggested that the supersensitivity was due to partial denervation of the bladder as a result of the obstruction, and that one consequence of this may be detrusor instability. The link between supersensitivity to ACh and detrusor overactivity is, however, not established. For example, Yokoyama et al. (1991) found that the responses to ACh of detrusor strips from patients with bladder instability were not significantly different from those without. The reasons for these conflicting results are unclear but may be partly explained by the fact that the denervation is "patchy", leaving parts of the detrusor with an intact innervation (Pandita et al. 2000).

The obstructed human bladder often shows an increased (up to $\approx$50%) atropine-resistant contractile component (Sjögren et al. 1982, Bayliss et al. 1999). This may be taken as indirect evidence of changes in the cholinergic functions of the bladder since normally, the atropine-resistant component is almost negligible (Andersson 1993, Tagliani et al. 1997, Bayliss et al. 1999).

Not only in the normal detrusor but also in the obstructed rat bladder M_3 receptors were found to play a predominant part in mediating detrusor contraction (Krichevsky et al. 1999). However, Braverman et al. (2002) showed that in rats, bladder outflow obstruction could change the muscarinic receptor subtype mediating bladder contraction from M_3 to M_2.

2.3.2   Detrusor overactivity

In obstructed bladders, and also in unstable human bladders (Charlton et al. 1999, Mills et al. 2000), areas within the detrusor may be more or less devoid of cholinergic nerves. A consequence of such a "patchy denervation" of the detrusor may be alterations of smooth muscle function, including increased coupling between individual cells. It has been suggested that such changes contribute to detrusor overactivity. However, when comparing detrusor strips from normal, idiopathic unstable, and hyperactive human bladders due to neurological damage, Kinder and Mundy (1987) found no significant differences in the degree of atropine inhibition of electrically induced contractions, and no significant differences in the concentration-response curves for ACh. Bayliss et al. (1999) showed atropine-resistant contractions in bladders from patients with idiopathic instability, a finding confirmed by O'Reilly et al. (2002). This suggests an increased importance of non-cholinergic mechanisms in the activation of the detrusor. In line with this, a decreased number of muscarinic receptors was found in overactive bladders without associated neurological disorders (Restorick and Mundy 1987).

2.3.3 Neurogenic bladders

Whether or not the muscarinic receptor functions are changed in neurogenic bladders has not been established. Lepor et al. (1989) found no age-related changes in muscarinic receptor density in normal or neurogenic bladders. In myelodysplastic bladders, Gup et al. (1989) found no super-sensitivity to carbachol and no changes in the binding properties of the muscarinic receptors. German et al. (1995), however, found that isolated detrusor strips from patients with detrusor hyperreflexia (neurogenic bladder dysfunction) were supersensitive to both carbachol and KCl but responded like normal controls to intramural nerve stimulation. The results were interpreted to suggest a state of postjunctional supersensitivity of the detrusor secondary to a partial parasympathetic denervation (German et al. 1995). An atropine-resistant component of the contraction of the human neurogenic bladder has been reported by some investigators (Saito et al. 1993), but not by others (Bayliss et al. 1999).

Compared with the normal bladder, the muscarinic subtype contribution to contraction in bladders with neurogenic damage may differ. In the denervated rat bladder (destruction of major pelvic ganglion and after spinal cord injury), M_2 receptors, or a combination of M_2 and M_3 mediated contractile responses (Braverman et al. 1998, 1999).

The muscarinic pre-junctional facilitatory mechanism seems to be upregulated in overactive bladders from chronic spinal cord transected rats. The facilitation in these preparations is primarily mediated by M_3 muscarinic receptors (Somogyi and de Groat 1999).

2.3.4 Diabetes

Voiding dysfunction is common in patients with diabetes mellitus, and a variety of urodynamic abnormalities may be found, including detrusor hyperreflexia (neurogenic bladder dysfunction) and impaired detrusor contractility (Kaplan et al. 1995). Bladders from diabetic animals showed increased density of muscarinic receptors and enhanced muscarinic receptor-mediated phosphoinositide hydrolysis (Latifpour et al. 1989, Mimata et al. 1995). An upregulation of the M_2 receptor mRNA has been reported in rats with streptozotocin-induced diabetes (Tong et al. 1999), and also a supersensitivity of postjunctional muscarinic receptors (Hashitani and Suzuki 1996). However, it is unclear what these receptor changes mean for the functional bladder disorders seen in diabetic patients. If found also in humans, they could contribute to voiding dysfunction and lower urinary tract symptoms. An aldose reductase inhibitor reduced the increase in muscarinic receptors and normalised the increased contractile response to ACh seen in rats with streptozotocin-induced diabetes (Kanda et al. 1997).

2.3.5 Aging and bladder effects of antimuscarinic drugs

The influence of age on muscarinic receptor density and sensitivity has been investigated in animal models, with partly conflicting results. Kolta et al. (1984) found that the bladder of aged rats seemed to develop an increased sensitivity to muscarinic receptor stimulation as a result of an increased number of muscarinic receptors. These results were not confirmed by Ordway et al. (1986) who found that an age-related increase in the responsiveness of the bladder could not be explained by a change in the number or affinity of muscarinic receptors. In contrast, Pagala et al. (2001) found a reduced response to bethanechol in aging rats, and suggested that this was the result of an age-related reduction in muscarinic receptors. Braverman et al. (2002) showed that in rats, aging could change the muscarinic receptor subtype mediating bladder contraction from M_3 to M_2, an observation that, if valid in humans, may have therapeutic implications.

Antimuscarinic drugs are active in the storage phase of the bladder, when there is normally no sacral parasympathetic outflow (de Groat et al. 1993, 1999). This suggests that during the storage phase, there is an ongoing stimulation of detrusor tone by ACh, most probably released from nerves. In fact, Yoshida et al. (2002) showed a basal ACh release in isolated human detrusor which is increased by stretching the muscle and by increasing tension. This release was age-dependent and significantly higher in bladders from old (>65 years) as compared to young (<65 years) patients. An increased local release of ACh could be expected to enhance the myogenic contractile activity of the detrusor, which seems to be increased in patients with detrusor overactivity (Brading 1997), and to increase afferent activity. If this is correct, inhibition of ACh release or blockade of the postjunctional muscarinic receptors should be expected to reduce bladder tone during storage, and to an increased bladder capacity. After administration of antimuscarinics to normal individuals as well as to patients with detrusor overactivity, such effects can be demonstrated (Andersson 1999).

The cause of an increased ACh release during storage can only be speculated on. Possibly, secondary to ischemic damage, damaged nerves may leak ACh (Brading 1997). Since focal denervation has been found as a characteristic of most disorders associated with detrusor overactivity, there may also be an increased postjunctional sensitivity to ACh in these disorders. Therapeutically, this should mean that it is more important to inhibit the postjunctional effects of ACh during storage than during voiding.

3.   Non-cholinergic mechanisms

In contrast to the normal human bladder, where contraction is almost exclusively mediated by ACh, a non-adrenergic, non-cholinergic (NANC) mechanism can be demonstrated in most animal species. NANC contractions have been reported to occur in normal human detrusor (Sjögren et al. 1982, Sibley 1984, Luheshi and Zar 1990, Ruggieri et al. 1990), but representing only a small proportion of the total contraction in response to nerve stimulation. In contrast, a significant NANC-mediated contraction (up to 40–50% of the total bladder contraction) has been demonstrated in morphologically and/or functionally changed human bladders and has been reported to occur in hypertrophic bladders (Sjögren et al. 1982, Smith and Chapple 1994, Bayliss et al. 1999, Calvert et al. 2001), idiopathic detrusor instability (Bayliss et al. 1999, O'Reilly et al. 2002), interstitial cystitis (Palea et al. 1993), neurogenic bladders (Wammack et al. 1995), and in the aging bladder (Yoshida et al. 2001). Good evidence shows that the transmitter responsible for the NANC component is ATP (Burnstock 2001).

Yoshida et al. (2001) investigated the contractile responses to KCl, carbachol, ATP, and electrical field stimulation, in human bladder specimens from three groups of patients undergoing cystectomy for bladder cancer. They were divided according to age into three groups: under 50 years, between 51 and 70 years, and over 70 years old. The contractile responses were not significantly different among the three groups. However, the atropine-sensitive and -resistant parts of contraction induced by electrical field stimulation were decreased and increased with age, respectively. Furthermore, significant positive and negative correlations were found between age and the purinergic, and age and the cholinergic neurotransmissions in human isolated bladder smooth muscle, respectively. The authors suggested that age-related changes in neurotransmissions may contribute to the changes in bladder function found in elderly people.

ATP acts on $P2X_1$ receptors in smooth muscle membranes of the detrusor (Lee et al. 2002, O'Reilly et al. 2001). However, other P2X receptor subtypes have been found in the bladder (Burnstock 2001). Urothelially released ATP, acting via $P2X_3$ receptors on a subpopulation of pelvic afferent fibres, may initiate activation of the bladder (Cockayne et al. 2000) and hypothetically induce detrusor overactivity, urge, frequency, and incontinence.

Moore et al. (2001) reported that detrusor from patients with idiopathic detrusor instability had a selective absence of $P2X_3$ and $P2X_5$ receptors and suggested that this specific lack might impair control of detrusor contractility and contribute to the pathophysiology of urge incontinence. However, O'Reilly et al. (2002) found in patients with idiopathic detrusor instability that $P2X_2$ receptors were significantly elevated, wheras other P2X receptor subtypes were significantly decreased. They reported that about 50% of the detrusor contraction in unstable bladders was purinergic, and they concluded that this abnormal purinergic transmission in the bladder might explain symptoms in these patients. They further suggested that the purinergic pathway could be a novel target for the pharmacological treatment of the overactive bladder.

4.   Closing remarks

If abnormalities in the purinergic transmission in the bladder can contribute to the symptoms of OAB, it is obvious that P2X receptors might be targets for pharmacological intervention. Abnormal purinergic activation of the detrusor may also explain why antimuscarinic treatment fails in a number of patients. Since there is an increased purinergic and a decreased cholinergic neurotransmission with age (Yoshida et al. 2001), this may be important when treating patients with detrusor overactivity. Whether or not this implies that drugs with combined effects on activation induced by muscarinic and purinergic receptors have better clinical effectiveness than drugs with only antimuscarinic activity, has to be demonstrated in randomised clinical trials.

5.   References

1. Abrams P, Cardozo L, Fall M, Griffiths D, Rosier P, Ulmsten U, van Kerrebroeck P, Victor A, Wein A (2002) The standardisation of terminology of lower urinary tract function: report from the Standardisation Sub-committee of the International Continence Society. Neurourol Urodyn 21(2): 167–178
2. Andersson K-E (1993) Pharmacology of lower urinary tract smooth muscles and penile erectile tissues. Pharmacol Rev 45(3): 253–308
3. Andersson K-E (1999) Advances in the pharmacological control of the bladder. Exp Physiol 84(1): 195–213
4. Andersson K-E (2002) Bladder activation: afferent mechanisms. Urology 59 [Suppl 5A]: 43–50
5. Andersson K-E, Appell R, Awad S, Chapple C, Drutz H, Fourcroy J, Finkbeiner A, Haab F, Wein A (2002) Pharmacological treatment of urinary incontinence. In: Abrams P, Khoury S, Wein A (eds) Incontinence, 2nd International Consultation on Incontinence. Plymbridge Distributors Ltd, UK: Plymouth, pp 489–511
6. Bayliss M, Wu C, Newgreen D, Mundy AR, Fry CH (1999) A quantitative study of atropine-resistant contractile responses in human detrusor smooth muscle, from stable, unstable and obstructed bladders. J Urol 162: 1833–1839
7. Bonev AD, Nelson MT (1993) Muscarinic inhibition of ATP-sensitive K+ channels by protein kinase C in urinary bladder smooth muscle. Am J Physiol 265: C1723–C1728
8. Brading AF (1997) A myogenic basis for the overactive bladder. Urology 50 [6A Suppl]: 57–67
9. Braverman A, Legos J, Young W, Luthin G, Ruggieri M (1999) M2 receptors in genito-urinary smooth muscle pathology. Life Sci 64: 429–436
10. Braverman AS, Karlovsky M, Pontari MA, Ruggieri MR (2002) Aging and hypertrophy change the muscarinic receptor subtypemediating contraction from M_3 to M_2. J Urol 167: 43 (abstract 170)

11. Braverman AS, Luthin GR, Ruggieri MR (1998) M2 muscarinic receptor contributes to contraction of the denervated rat urinary bladder. Am J Physiol 275: R1654–R1660

12. Burnstock G (2001) Purinergic signalling in lower urinary tract. In: Abbracchio MP, Williams M (eds) Handbook of experimental pharmacology, Vol 151/I Purinergic and pyrimidinergic signalling I. Molecular, nervous and urogenitary system function. Springer: Berlin, Heidelberg, pp 423–515

13. Calvert RC, Thompson CS, Khan MA, Mikhailidis DP, Morgan RJ, Burnstock G (2001) Alterations in cholinergic and purinergic signaling in a model of the obstructed bladder. J Urol 166(4): 1530–1533

14. Caulfield MP, Birdsall NJM (1998) International Union of Pharmacology. XVII. Classification of muscarinic acetylcholine receptors. Pharmacol Rev 50: 279–290

15. Charlton RG, Morley AR, Chambers P, Gillespie JI (1999) Focal changes in nerve, muscle and connective tissue in normal and unstable human bladder. BJU Int 84: 953–960

16. Cockayne DA, Hamilton SG, Zhu QM, Dunn PM, Zhong Y, Novakovic S, Malmberg AB, Cain G, Berson A, Kassotakis L, Hedley L, Lachnit WG, Burnstock G, McMahon SB, Ford AP (2000) Urinary bladder hyporeflexia and reduced pain-related behaviour in P2X3-deficient mice. Nature 407(6807): 1011–1015

17. D'Agostino G, Bolognesi ML, Lucchelli A, Vicini D, Balestra B, Spelta V, Melchiorre C, Tonini M (2000) Prejunctional muscarinic inhibitory control of acetylcholine release in the human isolated detrusor: involvement of the M4 receptor subtype. Br J Pharmacol 129: 493–500

18. de Groat WC, Booth AM, Yoshimura N (1993) Neurophysiology of micturition and its modification in animal models of human disease. In: Maggi CA (ed) The autonomic nervous system. Vol. 6, Chapter 8, Nervous control of the urogenital system. Harwood Academic Publishers: London, UK, pp 227–289

19. de Groat WC, Downie JW, Levin RM, Long Lin AT, Morrison JFB, Nishizawa O, Steers WD, Thor KB (1999) Basic neurophysiology and neuropharmacology. In: Abrams P, Khoury S, Wein A (eds) Incontinence, 1st International Consultation on Incontinence. Plymbridge Distributors Ltd: UK, pp 105–154

20. de Groat WC, Yoshimura N (2001) Pharmacology of the lower urinary tract. Annu Rev Pharmacol Toxicol 41: 691–721

21. Eglen RM, Choppin A, Watson N (2001) Therapeutic opportunities from muscarinic receptor research. Trends Pharmacol Sci 22: 409–414

22. German K, Bedwani J, Davies J, Brading AF, Stephenson TP (1995) Physiological and morphometric studies into the pathophysiology of detrusor hyperrflexia in neuropathic patients. J Urol 153: 1678–1683

23. Gosling JA, Gilpin SA, Dixon JS, Gilpin CJ (1986) Decrease in the autonomic innervation of human detrusor muscle in outflow obstruction. J Urol 136: 501–504

24. Gup DI, Baumann M, Lepor H, Shapiro E (1989) Muscarinic cholinergic receptors in normal pediatric and myelodysplastic bladders. J Urol 142: 595–599

25. Hald T, Horn T (1998) The human urinary bladder in ageing. Br J Urol 82 [Suppl 1]: 59–64

26. Harrison SCV, Hunnam GR, Farman P, Doyle PT (1987) Bladder instability and denervation in patients with bladder outflow obstruction. Br J Urol 60: 519–522

27. Hashitani H, Suzuki H (1996) Altered electrical properties of bladder smooth muscle in streptozotocin-induced diabetic rats. Br J Urol 77: 798–804

28. Hegde SS, Choppin A, Bonhaus D, Briaud S, Loeb M, Moy TM, Loury D, Eglen RM (1997) Functional role of M2 and M3 muscarinic receptors in the urinary bladder of rats in vitro and in vivo. Br J Pharmacol 120(8): 1409–1418

29. Hegde SS, Eglen RM (1999) Muscarinic receptor subtypes modulating smooth muscle contractility in the urinary bladder. Life Sci 64: 419–428

30. Kanda M, Eto K, Tanabe N, Sugiyama A, Hashimoto K, Ueno A (1997) Effects of ONO-2235, an aldose reductase inhibitor, on muscarinic receptors and contractile response of the urinary bladder in rats with streptozotocin-induced diabetes. Jpn J Pharmacol 73: 221–228

31. Kaplan SA, Te AE, Blaivas JG (1995) Urodynamic findings in patients with diabetic cystopathy. J Urol 153: 342–344

32. Kinder RB, Mundy AR (1987) Pathophysiology of idiopathic detrusor instability and detrusor hyperreflexia. An in vitro study of human detrusor muscle. Br J Urol 60: 509–515

33. Kolta MG, Wallace LJ, Gerald MC (1984) Age-related changes in sensitivity of rat urinary bladder to autonomic agents. Mech Ageing Dev 27(2): 183–188

34. Kotlikoff MI, Dhulipala P, Wang YX (1999) M2 signaling in smooth muscle cells. Life Sci 64: 437–442

35. Krichevsky VP, Pagala MK, Vaydovsky I, Damer V, Wise GJ (1999) Function of M3 muscarinic receptors in the rat urinary bladder following partial outlet obstruction. J Urol 161: 1644–1650

36. Latifpour J, Gousse A, Kondo S, Morita T, Weiss RM (1989) Effects of experimental diabetes on biochemical and functional characteristics of bladder muscarinic receptors. J Pharmacol Exp Ther 248: 81–88

37. Lee HY, Bardini M, Burnstock G (2000) Distribution of P2X receptors in the urinary bladder and the ureter of the rat. J Urol 163(6): 2002–2007

38. Lepor H, Gup D, Shapiro E, Baumann M (1989) Muscarinic cholinergic receptors in the normal and neurogenic human bladder. J Urol 142(3): 869–874

39. Luheshi GN, Zar MA (1990) Presence of non-cholinergic motor transmission in human isolated bladder. J Pharm Pharmacol 42(3): 223–224

40. Matsui M, Motomura D, Karasawa H, Fujikawa T, Jiang J, Komiya Y, Takahashi S, Taketo MM (2000) Multiple functional defects in peripheral autonomic organs in mice lacking muscarinic acetylcholine receptor gene for the M3 subtype. Proc Natl Acad Sci USA 97: 9579–9584

41. Mills IW, Greenland JE, McMurray G, McCoy R, Ho KM, Noble JG, Brading AF (2000) Studies of the pathophysiology of idiopathic detrusor instability: the physiological properties of the detrusor smooth muscle and its pattern of innervation. J Urol 163: 646–651

42. Milsom I, Abrams P, Cardozo L, Roberts RG, Thüroff J, Wein AJ (2001) How widespread are the symptoms of an overactive bladder and how are they managed? A population-based prevalence study. BJU Int 87(9): 760–766

43. Mimata H, Wheeler MA, Fukumoto Y, Takigawa H, Nishimoto T, Weiss RM, Latifpour J (1995) Enhancement of muscarinic receptor-coupled phosphatidyl inositol hydrolysis in diabetic bladder. Mol Cell Biochem 152: 71–76

44. Moore KH, Ray FR, Barden JA (2001) Loss of purinergic P2X(3) and P2X(5) receptor innervation in human detrusor from adults with urge incontinence. J Neurosci 21: RC166: 1–6

45. Ordway GA, Esbenshade TA, Kolta MG, Gerald MC, Wallace LJ (1986) Effect of age on cholinergic muscarinic responsiveness and receptors in the rat urinary bladder. J Urol 136(2): 492–496

46. O'Reilly BA, Kosaka AH, Chang TK, Ford AP, Popert R, McMahon SB (2001) A quantitative analysis of purinoceptor expression in the bladders of patients with symptomatic outlet obstruction. BJU Int 87(7): 617–622

47. O'Reilly BA, Kosaka AH, Chang TK, Ford AP, Popert R, Rymer JM, McMahon SB (2001) A quantitative analysis of purinoceptor expression in human fetal and adult bladders. J Urol 165(5): 1730–1734

48. O'Reilly BA, Kosaka AH, Knight GF, Chang TK, Ford AP, Rymer JM, Popert R, Burnstock G, McMahon SB (2002) P2X receptors and their role in female idiopathic detrusor instability. J Urol 167(1): 157–164

49. Palea S, Artibani W, Ostardo E, Trist DG, Pietra C (1993) Evidence for purinergic neurotransmission in human urinary bladder affected by interstitial cystitis. J Urol 150: 2007–2012

50. Pagala MK, Tetsoti L, Nagpal D, Wise GJ (2001) Aging effects on contractility of longitudinal and circular detrusor and trigone of rat bladder. J Urol 166(2): 721–727

51. Pandita RK, Fujiwara M, Alm P, Andersson K-E (2000) Cystometric evaluation of bladder function in non-anesthetized mice with and without bladder outlet obstruction. J Urol 164(4): 1385–1389

52. Restorick JM, Mundy AR (1987) The density of cholinergic and alpha and beta adrenergic receptors in the normal and hyper-reflexic human detrusor. Br J Urol 63: 32–35

53. Ruggieri MR, Whitmore KE, Levin RM (1990) Bladder purinergic receptors. J Urol 144(1): 176–181

54. Saito M, Kondo A, Kato T, Miyake K (1993) Response of the human neurogenic bladder induced by intramural nerve stimulation. Nippon Hinyokika Gakkai Zasshi 84: 507–513

55. Sibley GN (1984) A comparison of spontaneous and nerve-mediated activity in bladder muscle from man, pig and rabbit. J Physiol (Lond) 354: 431–443

56. Sibley GN (1987) The physiological response of the detrusor muscle to experimental bladder outflow obstruction in the pig. Br J Urol 60: 332–336

57. Sjögren C, Andersson K-E, Husted S, Mattiasson A, Møller-Madsen B (1982) Atropine resistance of the transmurally stimulated isolated human bladder. J Urol 128: 1368–1371

58. Smith DJ, Chapple CR (1994) In vitro response of human bladder smooth muscle in unstable obstructed male bladders: a study of pathophysiological causes? Neurourol Urodyn 134: 14–15

59. Somogyi GT, de Groat WC (1992) Evidence for inhibitory nicotinic and facilitatory muscarinic receptors in cholinergic nerve terminals of the rat urinary bladder. J Auton Nerv Syst 37: 89–97

60. Somogyi GT, de Groat WC (1999) Function, signal transduction mechanisms and plasticity of presynaptic muscarinic receptors in the urinary bladder. Life Sci 64: 411–418

61. Speakman MJ, Brading AF, Gilpin CJ, Dixon JS, Gilpin SA, Gosling JA (1987) Bladder outflow obstruction – a cause of denervation supersensitivity. J Urol 138: 1461–1466

62. Tagliani M, Candura SM, Di Nucci A, Franceschetti GP, D'Agostino G, Ricotti P, Fiori E, Tonini M (1997) A re-appraisal of the nature of the atropine-resistant contraction to electrical field stimulation in the human isolated detrusor muscle. Naunyn Schmiedebergs Arch Pharmacol 356: 750–755

63. Tobin G, Sjögren C (1998) Prejunctional facilitatory and inhibitory modulation of parasympathetic nerve transmission in the rabbit urinary bladder. J Autonom Nerv Syst 68:153–156

64. Tong YC, Chin WT, Cheng JT (1999) Alterations in urinary bladder M2-muscarinic receptor protein and mRNA in 2-week streptozotocin-induced diabetic rats. Neurosci Lett 277: 173–176
65. Wammack R, Weihe E, Dienes H-P, Hohenfellner R (1995) Die neurogene Blase in vitro. Akt Urol 26: 16–18
66. Yamanishi T, Chapple CR, Chess-Williams R (2001) Which muscarinic receptor is important in the bladder? World J Urol 19: 299–306
67. Yamanishi T, Chapple CR, Yasuda K, Chess-Williams R (2002) The role of M2 muscarinic receptor subtypes in mediating contraction of the pig bladder base after cyclic adenosine monophosphate elevation and/or selective M3 inactivation. J Urol 167: 397–401
68. Yokoyama O, Nagano K, Kawaguchi K, Hisazumi H (1991) The response of the detrusor muscle to acetylcholine in patients with infravesical obstruction. Urol Res 19: 117–121
69. Yoshida M, Inadome A, Murakami S, Miyamae K, Iwashita H, Otani M, Masunaga K, Miyamoto Y, Ueda S (2002) Effects of age and muscle stretching on acetylcholine release in isolated human bladder smooth muscle. J Urol 167: 40 (abstract 160)
70. Yoshida M, Homma Y, Inadome A, Yono M, Seshita H, Miyamoto Y, Murakami S, Kawabe K, Ueda S (2001) Age-related changes in cholinergic and purinergic neurotransmission in human isolated bladder smooth muscles. Exp Gerontol 36: 99–109

Correspondence address: K-E Andersson, MD, PhD, Department of Clinical Pharmacology, Institute for Laboratory Medicine, Lund University Hospital, S-221 85 Lund, Sweden (E-mail: Karl-Erik.Andersson@klinfarm.lu.se).

Changes in the receptor profile of the lower urinary tract in the aging male

C. Hampel, P. C. Dolber, C. M. Kuhn,
D. A. Schwinn, K. B. Thor, and *J. W. Thüroff*

Department of Urology, Johannes Gutenberg University Mainz,
Mainz, Germany

Contents

1.   Introduction

Benign prostatic hyperplasia (BPH) is one of the most common effects of aging in men. Epidemiologists estimate that about one quarter of all men over 50 years of age suffer from BPH-derived voiding symptoms. Future demographic developments, with higher relative shares of older people, will increase the socioeconomic impact of this disease. Polder et al. (1994) calculated for the Netherlands that the treatment costs of BPH will double by 2035. Office visits for BPH related symptoms increased in the USA from 1.4 million in 1990 to 6 million in 1995, reflecting the increased public awareness of the problem and the increased desire for treatment (Kaplan et al. 1996).

Lower urinary tract symptoms (LUTS) associated with bladder outlet obstruction (BOO) caused by BPH can be subdivided into "obstructive" and "irritative" symptoms. Whereas obstructive symptoms – weak stream, post-void dribbling and formation of post-void residual (PVR) – are the main issues of interest in the follow-up of BPH treatment in response to pharmacological or surgical treatment of the prostate, patients complain predominantly about irritative symptoms such as nocturia, frequency, and urgency. According to Seaman et al., three of the four most bothersome symptoms of BPH are irritative (Seaman et al. 1994) (Fig. 1). The patho-physiology behind irritative BOO symptoms is detrusor hyperactivity. Urodynamically, detrusor hyperactivity results in uninhibited detrusor

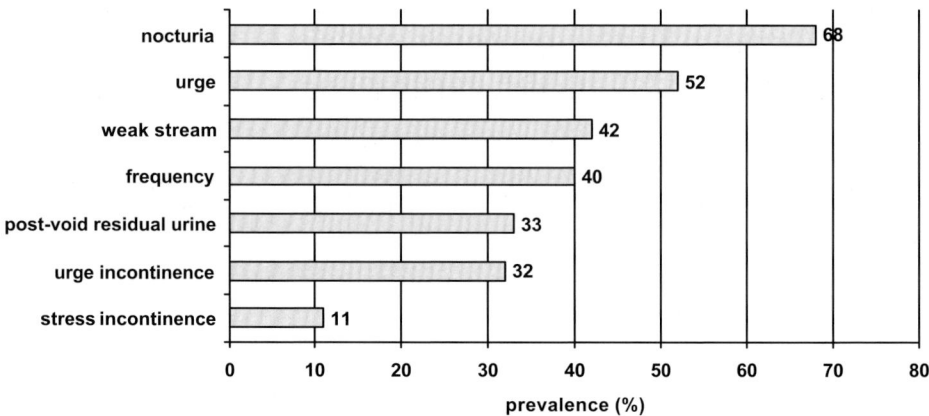

Fig. 1. Prevalence of BOO-associated LUTS in BPH patients (Seaman et al. 1994)

contractions, which are even more common in patients with BPH than urodynamically defined obstruction, i.e. low voiding flow associated with high detrusor pressure (Seaman et al. 1994). Irritative symptoms in BPH patients are thought to be a consequence of the detrusor smooth muscle cell hypertrophy that accompanies the increased work required to overcome the elevated bladder outlet resistance (Chapple et al. 1994, Cucchi 1991, Gosling and Dixon 1983, Uvelius et al. 1984). The resulting detrusor instability even seems to be an energy saving mechanism of the bladder to optimise bladder depletion (Cucchi 1991, Cucchi et al. 1997).

Despite the fact that low urine flow or a weak stream are neither the most prevalent nor the most bothersome symptoms for BPH patients (Kaplan et al. 1996), most studies of prostate ablation focus on urine flow measurements to assess therapeutic success (Cummings et al. 1995, Javle et al. 1996). Abrams et al. evaluated the postoperative symptom relief of BPH patients after TUR-P. Their results showed a symptom relief of 90% for obstructive symptoms such as weak stream. However, every second BPH patient continued to report persistent irritative symptoms (Abrams et al. 1979) (Fig. 2). Relief of irritative BPH symptoms is more difficult, less effective, and takes more time than the relief of obstructive symptoms (Neal 1994, Neal et al. 1989). In other words, clinical observations of BPH patients have found continued irritative symptoms even after effective removal of the obstruction with subsequent normalization of flow rates. This indicates an indirect and longlasting enhancement of bladder contractility (Chai et al. 1999, Hakenberg 1999).

One possibility for enhanced bladder contractility after BOO is an altered $\alpha 1$-adrenergic receptor profile on the detrusor smooth muscle cells. The pathophysiological hypothesis of rising $\alpha 1$-adrenergic bladder susceptibility postulates the bladder recruitment of all possible expulsive forces under circumstances of increased outlet resistance to improve contractility and emptying effectiveness. This theory is supported by reports showing decreased detrusor irritability by alpha-sympatholytics (Steers et al. 1994).

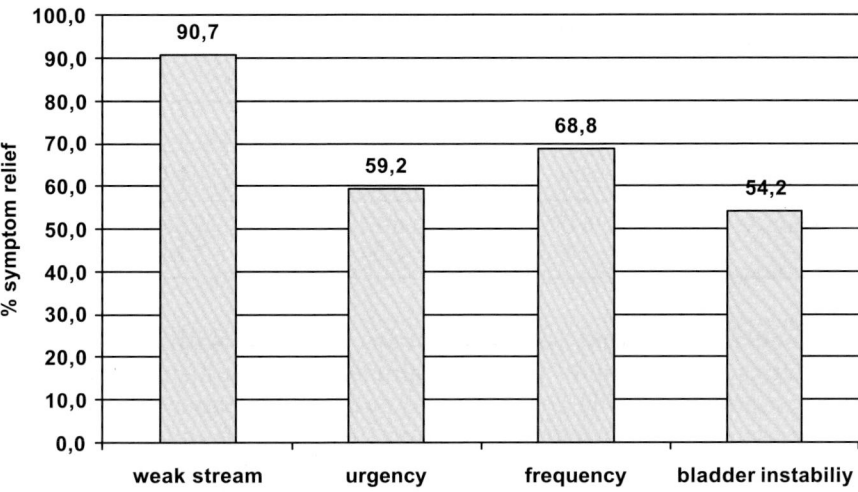

Fig. 2. Symptom relief of BOO-associated LUTS in BPH patients after transurethral resection of the prostate (Abrams et al. 1979)

2. Classification and subtypes of adrenergic receptors

When Ahlquist described the first subdivision of adrenergic receptors into α and β receptors in Ahlquist 1948, he referred to differences in potency of various agonists. The discovery of pre- and postsynaptical α-receptor subtypes led to the classification of α1- and α2-adrenoceptors in 1974 (Langer 1974, Starke et al. 1974). Most recently, molecular cloning techniques and pharmacological binding studies have shown a subset of 3 α1-adrenergic receptor (AR) clones, named α1a (formerly known as α1c), α1b, and α1d (formerly known as α1a or α1a/d) (Table 1) with different mRNA sequences (Bruno et al. 1991, Cotecchia et al. 1988, Lomasney et al. 1991, Perez et al. 1991, Ramarao et al. 1992, Schwinn et al. 1990, Voigt et al. 1990) and different affinity profiles towards their natural agonists norepinephrine and epinephrine (Faure et al. 1994) (Table 2). These three receptor clones show unique expression patterns for different tissues (for example, α1a $= \alpha$1d $> \alpha$1b in prostate tissue, α1a $\gg \alpha$1b $\gg \alpha$1d in heart tissue) (Langer 1999).

Table 1. Historical and new nomenclature of α1 AR subtypes

Native	Clone (historical nomenclature)	Clone (new nomenclature)
α_{1A}	α_{1c}	α_{1a}
α_{1B}	α_{1b}	α_{1b}
α_{1D}	$\alpha_{1a}, \alpha_{1d}, \alpha_{1a/d}$	α_{1d}

Table 2. Affinity of norepinephrine and epinephrine towards α1a, α1b and α1d adrenergic receptors (negative logarithm of half maximal binding concentration in mol/l)[37]

Compound	pKi		
	α1a	α1b	α1d
Norepinephrine	6.0	6.15	7.36
Epinephrine	6.3	6.54	7.24

The popular treatment of obstructive patients with α1-selective sympatholytics (for example, prazosin, alfuzosin, tamsulosin) targets the dynamic component of BPH and decreases outflow resistance by relaxation of the prostatic smooth muscle fibres (Caine 1990, Ruffolo and Hieble 1999). Since α1a and α1d AR are the predominant isoforms in the prostate, the α1a/d selective compound tamsulosin is called "uroselective", with particular reference to α1a selectivity (Beique et al. 1998, de Mey 1999, Debruyne and Van der Poel 1999, Martin et al. 1997, Na et al. 1998). Interestingly, compared with tamsulosin, which proved to relieve obstructive as well as irritative symptoms, the highly α1a-selective compound RS-17053 shows less activity in vitro with respect to inhibition of lower urinary tract contractility (urethra, prostate, bladder neck) (Kenny et al. 1996).

However, the rapid onset of the relief of irritative symptoms in BPH patients treated with α1 adrenergic antagonists (Caine 1990) cannot be explained by regression of detrusor hypertrophy and secondary changes but imply a direct effect of the α1-antagonist on the unstable detrusor. Moreover, in animal studies with mechanically generated entirely static outlet obstruction (where α1-antagonists cannot influence the degree of obstruction by decreasing any dynamic muscular constriction), prazosin was still effective in reducing urinary frequency (Steers et al. 1994). Finally, Persson et al. reported an increased nerve growth factor (NGF) production in smooth muscle fibres that are mechanically stretched, as occurs during bladder outlet obstruction (Persson et al. 1995). NGF is known to cause particularly proliferation of adrenergic innervation (Steers et al. 1996).

All these findings led to the hypothesis of an involvement of increased alpha-adrenergic detrusor susceptibility in evolving irritative symptoms during the course of bladder outlet obstruction.

3. Material and methods

To elucidate the potential role of changes in the α1 adrenergic susceptibility of the obstructed bladder, we established a rat model of bladder outlet obstruction with subsequent detrusor hypertrophy and hyperactivity. Only female nulliparous age-matched Sprague-Dawley rats (175–200 g) were used to avoid obstruction of ductus deferentis and seminal vesicles with consecutive ascending infections in case of distal ligation of a male urethra.

Micturition behaviour of the animals was monitored before and after obstruction in metabolism cages with computer assistance. Sympathetic detrusor innervation was measured by immunohistochemistry, using monoclonal anti-dopamin-β-hydroxylase-antibodies and fluorescent secondary antibodies. Neurotransmitter bioavailability (norepinephrine and epinephrine) was quantified by high performance liquid chromatography (HPLC) of detrusor tissue. We investigated the regional gene expression of all three $\alpha 1$ adrenergic receptor (AR) subtypes in normal and obstructed rat bladders by using a quantitative competitive reverse transcriptase polymerase chain reaction (C-RT-PCR) technique. Afterwards, a comparison of the total $\alpha 1$ AR mRNA expression with the total $\alpha 1$ AR membrane protein content determined by [^{125}I]HEAT saturation binding was performed in order to investigate the possible post-transcriptional modifications of $\alpha 1$ AR protein translation during bladder outlet obstruction. Finally, the in vitro contractility of bladder strips derived from unobstructed control rats and obstructed animals was investigated in the organ bath laboratory.

4. Results

4.1 Micturition behaviour

After six weeks of obstruction, the average bladder mass increased by 600% (Fig. 3). This increase was consistent throughout different obstruction series several months apart.

The computer assisted long term-observation of the micturition behaviour of the Sprague-Dawley rats was able to show the occurrence of irritative voiding symptoms in the course of bladder outlet obstruction. Moreover, comparing sham operated animals with unoperated control animals, the surgical intervention itself could be excluded as a confounding factor. No difference was found in the micturition behaviour between sham operated and control animals with respect to bladder weight, micturition volume per voiding event per body mass and micturition frequency per body mass. However, obstructed animals showed a completely different micturition behaviour. By using certain cut-off values for micturition volume per voiding event per body mass (0.3 ml/200 g) and micturition frequency per body mass (1.9/200 g/h) it was possible to discriminate between obstructed and unobstructed rats with 100% specificity and sensitivity. The increase of micturition frequency and the decrease of the urine volume per void was highly significant (Figs. 4, 5).

4.2 Immunohistochemistry

When using immunohistochemical staining procedures for sympathetic nerve fibres, perivascular sympathetic nerves have to be differentiated from detrusor associated nerves. Since both types of nerves provide the same immunofluorescence, the detrusor associated nerve fibre density of the

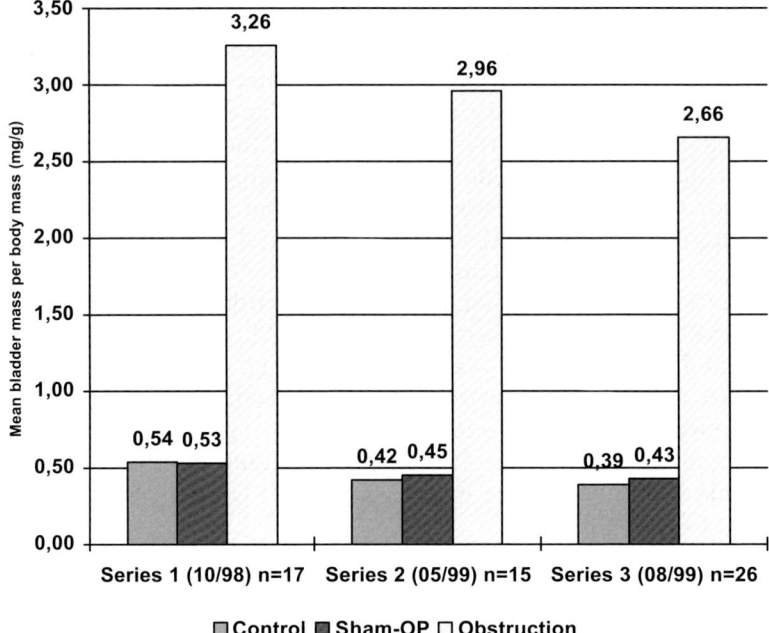

Fig. 3. Mean bladder mass per body mass of age-matched Sprague-Dawley rats 6 weeks after obstruction or sham operation

bladder sections had to be calculated without the use of computer assisted image analysis. The detrusor sections of obstructed rats showed a marked reduction in sympathetic nerve fibre density of about 80%, although one has to keep in mind the average increase in total bladder weight of about 600% (Fig. 6). In conclusion, the total number of nerve fibres per whole organ increased, but the increase was to small as to compensate detrusor hypertrophy, thus leading to a reduced neurotransmitter bioavailability.

The HPLC of detrusor tissue for evaluation of the sympathetic neurotransmitter concentration provided results comparable to the immunohistochemical findings. Although the absolute amount of norepinephrine and epinephrine per whole bladder increased, the relative tissue concentration decreased due to the enormous detrusor hypertrophy (Figs. 7, 8). Thus, the changed neurotransmitter bioavailability in obstructed rats cannot directly explain the bladder irritability and hyperactivity that was observed during the micturition behaviour recordings.

4.3 Receptor profiles

When tissue RNA was extracted from several bladders of each group (unoperated control, sham operated control, and obstructed), no statistical difference was found in $\alpha 1$ AR mRNA content between sham operated and unoperated control tissue. Therefore, their data were pooled, and the pooled

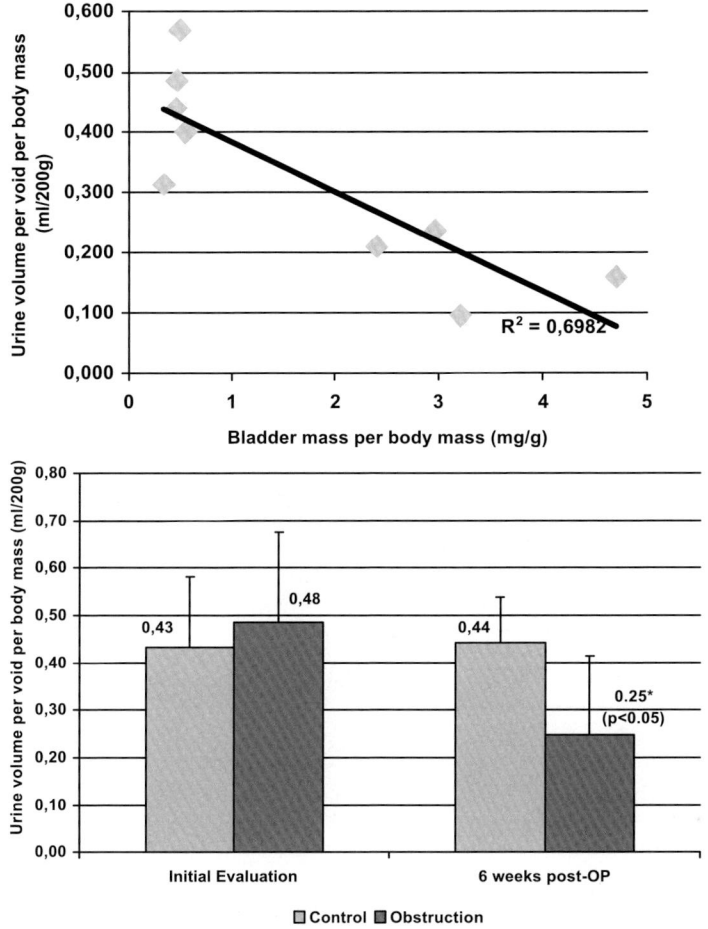

Fig. 4. Correlation between mean urine volume per micturition event per body mass and bladder mass per body mass (above); mean urine volume per micturition event per body mass before and 6 weeks after obstruction (below) (error bars reflect the standard deviation from the mean)

group was defined as the "control" group. Each region of the bladder (trigone, midbody, dome) was investigated separately.

Surprisingly, no trigone to detrusor gradient was found in the expression levels of α1a, α1b and α1d AR mRNA in detrusor from either controls or obstructed animals as might be expected based on classical literature (Wein and Levin 1979). In other words, trigone, midbody, and dome all contained similar amounts of α1 AR mRNA in each group (Fig. 9).

In detrusor tissue from control animals, there was a marked preponderance of the α1a AR mRNA as previously reported (Scofield et al. 1995). α1d AR mRNA was detected at levels approximately 1/3 those of the α1a AR mRNA subtype. The α1b AR mRNA was found only in very small amounts (<10% of the concentrations of the α1a AR mRNA) (Fig. 9).

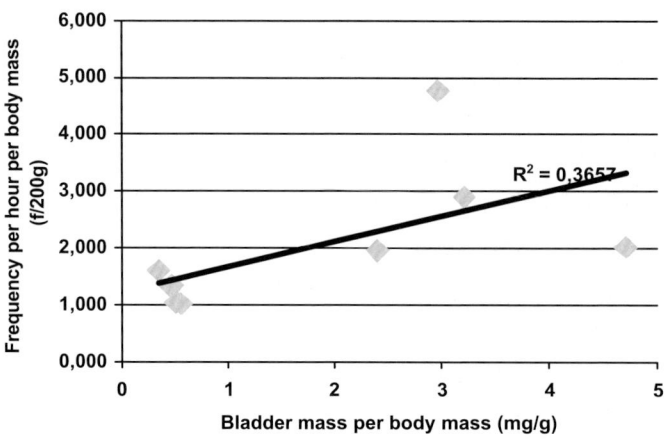

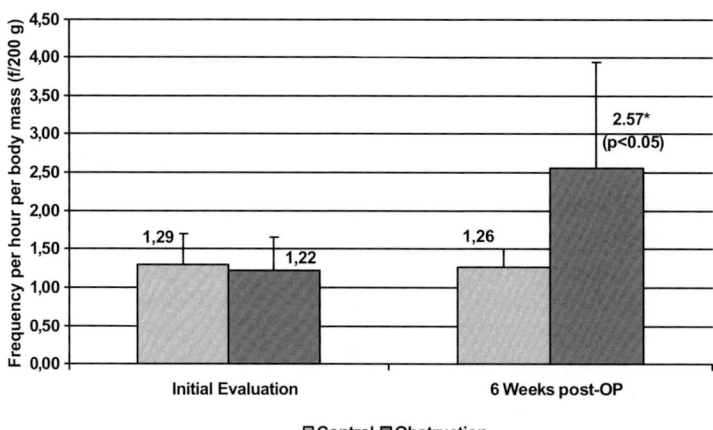

Fig. 5. Correlation between frequency per hour per body mass and bladder mass per body mass (above); mean frequency per hour per body mass before and 6 weeks after obstruction (below) (error bars reflect the standard deviation from the mean)

In contrast to the control animals, detrusor tissue from obstructed animals contained predominantly α1d AR mRNA, the subtype that is virtually absent in other tissues, such as heart or vascular tissue (Fig. 10).

The comparison of the total α1 AR mRNA expression in detrusor tissue with its α1-adrenoceptor membrane protein content determined by [^{125}I]HEAT saturation binding studies showed no significant differences in the ratios between mRNA expression and subsequent protein translation (Fig. 11). That indicates a similar efficiency of protein translation from mRNA templates for both, normal and obstructed detrusor cells.

4.4 Contractility studies

The in vitro contractility studies of obstructed and normal bladder strips showed a qualitatively different response to contractility modulation by

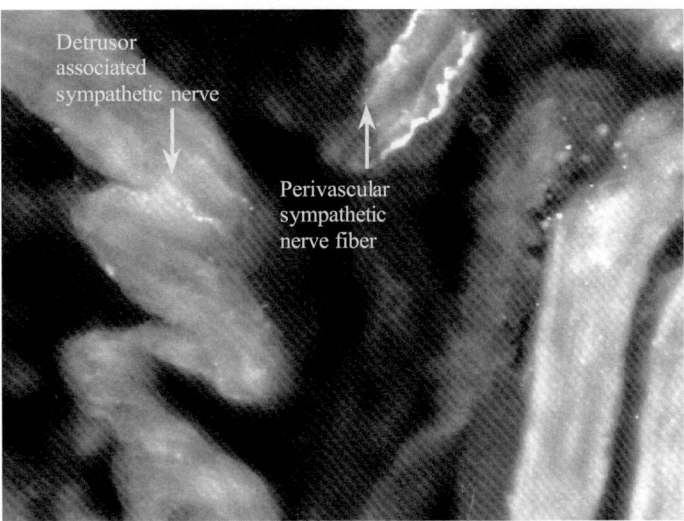

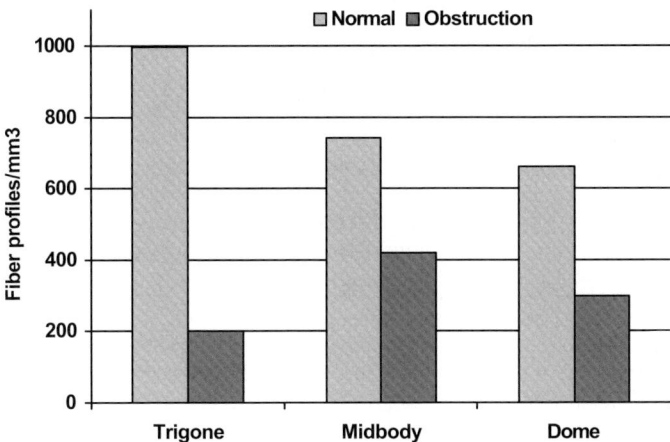

Fig. 6. Fluorescence micrograph of a 20 μm section of detrusor muscle (immunohistochemical anti-DBH-staining, magnification × 1000); perivascular and detrusor associated nerve fibres are shown side by side and elucidate the impossibility of computer-assisted image analysis for quantification of detrusor associated sympathetic nerve fibre density. The data are derived from a hand count of sympathetic nerve fibres

sympathetic agonists and antagonists. Obstructed and normal bladder strips developed spontaneous activity with characteristic amplitude and frequency on top of a baseline tension. These phasic contractions could be modulated by addition of norepinephrine in a dose-dependent fashion and was compared with a control strip without any norepinephrine stimulation. Obstructed bladder strips showed a increased contractility after norepinephrine stimulation, whereas the spontaneous activity of normal detrusor

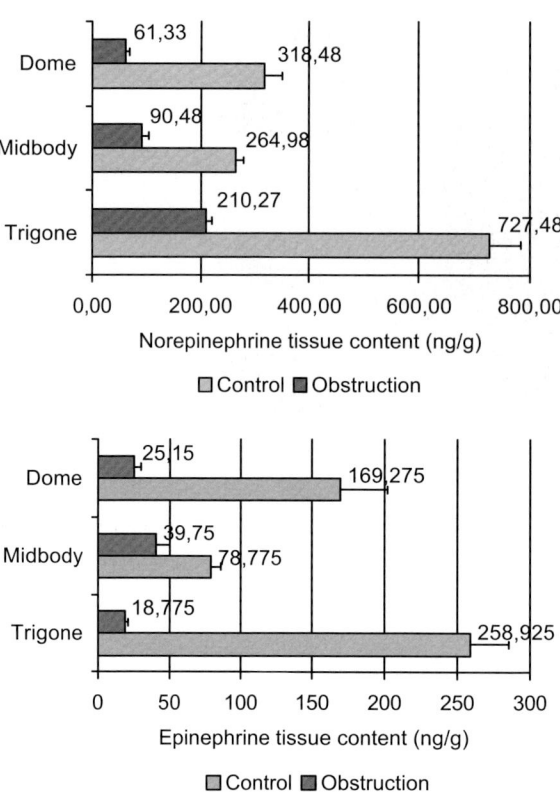

Fig. 7. Norepinephrine and epinephrine tissue concentrations (measured by HPLC) reflect the sympathetic neurotransmitter bioavailability and match the immuno-histochemical findings of nerve fibre density

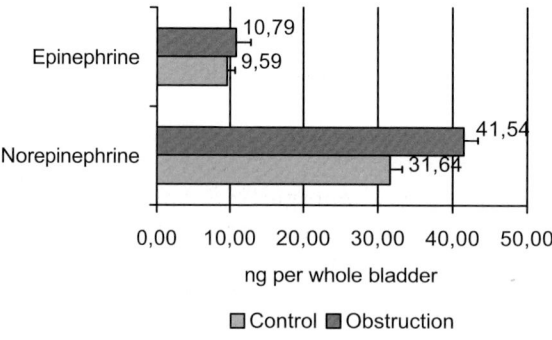

Fig. 8. Norepinephrine and epinephrine tissue contents (measured by HPLC) per whole bladder reflect the sympathetic neuroplasticity (nerve sprouting) and match the immunohistochemical findings of total nerve fibre number per bladder

strips diminished and the baseline tension lowered (Fig. 12). The relaxation of the normal bladder strips can be explained by a β-sympathomimetic effect, whereas the increased contractility of obstructed strips represents a

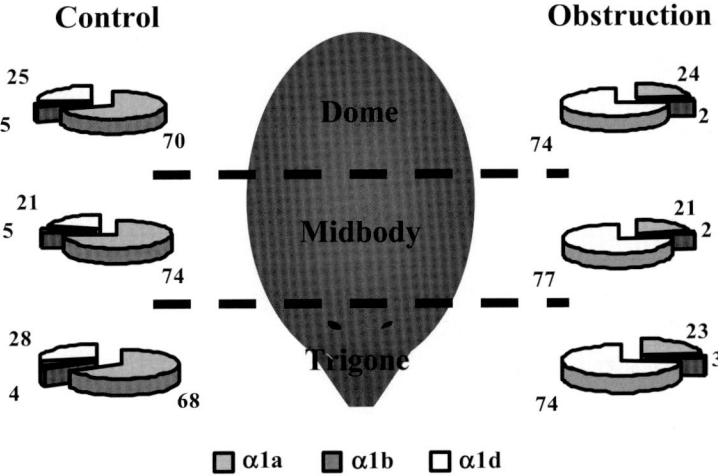

Fig. 9. Regional relative subtype share of $\alpha 1$ AR subtypes in rat detrusor as derived from quantitative competitive RT-PCR

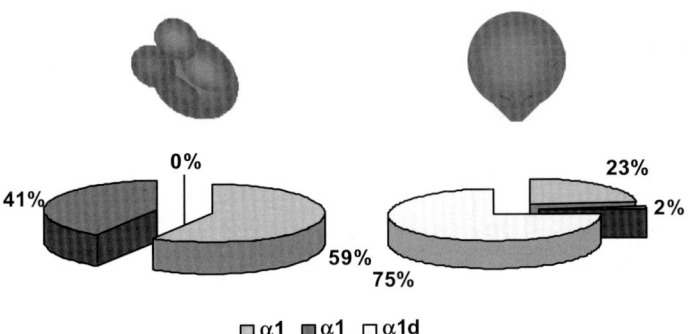

Fig. 10. Regional relative subtype share of $\alpha 1$ AR subtypes in rat detrusor and heart muscle as derived from quantitative competitive RT-PCR

$\alpha 1$-sympathomimetic effect due to either an increased $\alpha 1$-adrenergic detrusor susceptibility or a decreased α-adrenergic influence. This was proven by using the $\alpha 1$-selective sympathomimetic compound phenylephrine as the response to $\alpha 1$ adrenergic stimulation was much more pronounced in obstructed strips than in normal strips (Fig. 13). Hence, increased $\alpha 1$ adrenergic detrusor susceptibility of obstructed bladder strips may reflect the functional effect of the molecular changes in $\alpha 1$ adrenergic receptor subtype distribution.

5.   Discussion and conclusion

The rat model of bladder outlet obstruction provided many interesting results that may be able to elucidate the origin of BPH related irritative

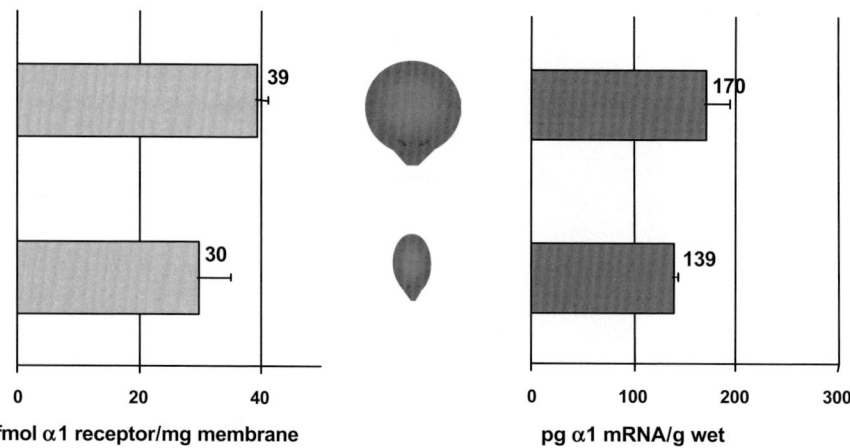

Fig. 11. Comparison between total α1 AR mRNA expression and receptor protein translation in obstructed and normal detrusor tissue as derived from quantitative competitive RT-PCR and [125I]HEAT saturation binding studies

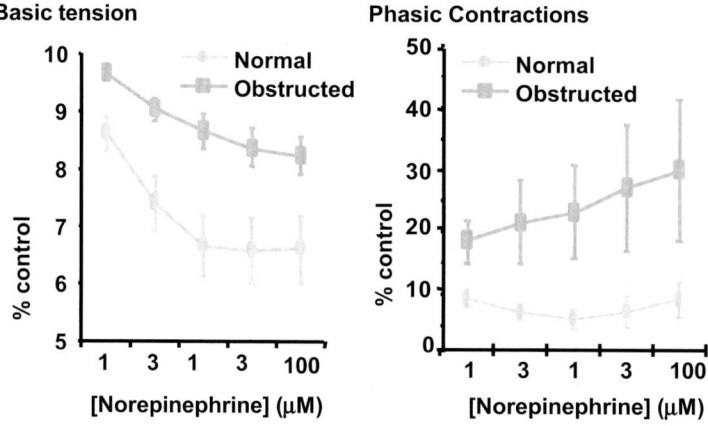

Fig. 12. In vitro contractility of detrusor strips of obstructed and normal control rats with respect to norepinephrine modulation of spontaneous activity (error bars reflect standard deviation from the mean)

LUTS – one of the most bothersome conditions of aging men. Our data are conclusive and explain the above mentioned clinical observations in BPH patients. However, overinterpretation of the results has to be avoided, and much more research is needed to be able to transfer these findings from the animal model to humans. Recently, Lluel et al. reported an increased α1-adrenergic detrusor susceptibility in older Wistar rats (30 months) compared with younger control animals (10 months) (Lluel et al. 2000) (Fig. 14). This may be another hint that modulation of the α1 adrenergic receptor profile is an important principle of the development of irritative LUTS in the course of aging, whether symptoms are obstruction derived or not.

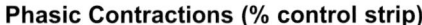
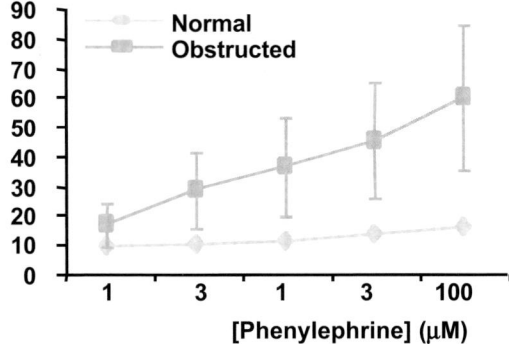

Phasic Contractions (% control strip)

Fig. 13. In vitro contractility of detrusor strips of obstructed and normal control rats with respect to phenylephrine modulation of spontaneous activity (error bars reflect standard deviation from the mean)

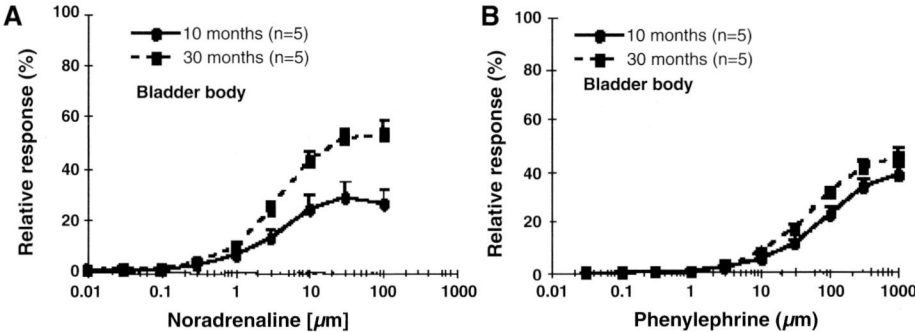

Fig. 14. In vitro contractility of detrusor strips of young (10 months) and older (30 months) Wistar rats with respect to norepinephrine and phenylephrine modulation of 80 mM KCl-provoked activity (Lluel et al. 2000)

Although it still has to be determined to what degree the increased alpha-adrenergic detrusor susceptibility contributes to the evolving irritative symptoms of BOO, one may speculate about the usefulness of various $\alpha 1$-antagonists in the treatment of maintained bladder irritability after effectively removed obstruction. $\alpha 1$-blockers, especially $\alpha 1d$ selective compounds, may be able to replace antimuscarinics (for example, oxybutinin) due to minor side effects. $\alpha 1a$-selective drugs would not be favourable for this indication, since the expected side effects would include $\alpha 1a$ excitation of heart and vessel receptor isoforms with consecutive hypotension. Moreover, these compounds would not target the predominant receptor subtype of the unstable detrusor. An $\alpha 1d$-selective antagonist like BMY 7378 seems to be promising for further investigations, since it is expected to cause less cardiovascular side effects than the $\alpha 1a/d$ selective

Table 3. Affinity of various α1-antagonists towards α1a, α1b and α1d adrenergic receptors (negative logarithm of half maximal binding concentration in mol/l)

Compound	pKi		
	α1a	α1b	α1d
Prazosin (Faure et al. 1994)	9.77	9.60	10.18
Tamsulosin (Foglar et al. 1995)	10.5	9.2	10.0
RS 17053 (Kenny et al. 1996)	8.6	7.3	7.1
BMY 7378 (Wetzel et al. 1995)	6.6	7.2	9.4

tamsulosin without losing inhibition potency regarding the target organ (Table 3).

6.　References

1. Abrams PH, Farrar DJ, Turner-Warwick RT, Whiteside CG, Feneley RC (1979) The results of prostatectomy: a symptomatic and urodynamic analysis of 152 patients. J Urol 121: 640–642
2. Ahlquist RP (1948) A study of the adrenotropic receptors. Am J Physiol 153: 586–600
3. Beique L, Por CP, Evans MF (1998) Are the new selective alpha-blockers better than non-selective alpha-blockers for benign prostatic hyperplasia? Can Fam Physician 44: 2659–2662
4. Bruno JF, Whittaker J, Song JF, Berelowitz M (1991) Molecular cloning and sequencing of a cDNA encoding a human alpha 1A adrenergic receptor. Biochem Biophys Res Commun 179: 1485–1490
5. Caine M (1990) Alpha-adrenergic blockers for the treatment of benign prostatic hyperplasia. Urol Clin North Am 17: 641–649
6. Chai TC, Gemalmaz H, Andersson KE, Tuttle JB, Steers WD (1999) Persistently increased voiding frequency despite relief of bladder outlet obstruction. J Urol 161: 1689–1693
7. Chapple CR, Burt RP, Andersson PO, Greengrass P, Wyllie M, Marshall I (1994) Alpha 1-adrenoceptor subtypes in the human prostate. Br J Urol 74: 585–589
8. Cotecchia S, Schwinn DA, Randall RR, Lefkowitz RJ, Caron MG, Kobilka BK (1988) Molecular cloning and expression of the cDNA for the hamster alpha 1-adrenergic receptor. Proc Natl Acad Sci USA 85: 7159–763
9. Cucchi A (1991) Dynamics of micturition in benign prostatic hypertrophy patients with compensated obstruction of the vesical outlet: a denervation supersensitivity-related energy-saving mechanism. J Urol 146: 1348–1351
10. Cucchi A, Achilli MP, Ravasi S, Arrigoni N (1997) Detrusor instability as an energy-saving device in prostatic obstruction. J Urol 157: 866–870
11. Cummings JM, Parra RO, Boullier JA (1995) Laser prostatectomy: initial experience and urodynamic follow-up. Urology 45: 414–418
12. de Mey C (1999) alpha(1)-Blockers for Bph: are there differences? Eur Urol 36 [Suppl S3]: 52–63
13. Debruyne FM, Van der Poel HG (1999) Clinical experience in Europe with uroselective alpha1-antagonists. Eur Urol 36 [Suppl] 1: 54–58

14. Faure C, Pimoule C, Vallancien G, Langer SZ, Graham D (1994) Identification of alpha 1-adrenoceptor subtypes present in the human prostate. Life Sci 54: 1595–1605
15. Foglar R, Shibata K, Horie K, Hirasawa A, Tsujimoto G (1995) Use of recombinant alpha 1-adrenoceptors to characterize subtype selectivity of drugs for the treatment of prostatic hypertrophy. Eur J Pharmacol 288: 201–207
16. Gosling JA, Dixon JS (1983) Detrusor morphology in relation to bladder outlet obstruction and instability. Benign Prostatic Hypertrophy. Verlag Publisher: Berlin, pp 666–671
17. Hakenberg OW, Pinnock CB, Marshall VR (1999) The follow-up of patients with unfavourable early results of transurethral prostatectomy. BJU Int 84: 799–804
18. Javle P, Jenkins SA, West C, Parsons KF (1996) Quantification of voiding dysfunction in patients awaiting transurethral prostatectomy. J Urol 156: 1014–1819
19. Kaplan SA, Bowers DL, Te AE, Olsson CA (1996) Differential diagnosis of prostatism: A 12-year retrospective analysis of symptoms, urodynamics and satisfaction with therapy. J Urol 155: 1305–1308
20. Kenny BA, Miller AM, Williamson IJ, J OC, Chalmers DH, Naylor AM (1996) Evaluation of the pharmacological selectivity profile of alpha 1 adrenoceptor antagonists at prostatic alpha 1 adrenoceptors: binding, functional and in vivo studies. Br J Pharmacol 118: 871–878
21. Langer SZ (1974) Presynaptic regulation of catecholamine release. Biochem Pharmacol 23: 1793–1800
22. Langer SZ (1999) History and nomenclature of alpha1-adrenoceptors. Eur Urol 36 [Suppl] 1: 2–6
23. Lluel P, Palea S, Barras M, et al (2000) Functional and morphological modifications of the urinary bladder in aging female rats. Am J Physiol Regul Integr Comp Physiol 278: R964–R972
24. Lomasney JW, Cotecchia S, Lorenz W, Leung WY, Schwinn DA, Yang-Feng TL, Brownstein M, Lefkowitz RJ, Caron MG (1991) Molecular cloning and expression of the cDNA for the alpha 1A-adrenergic receptor. The gene for which is located on human chromosome 5. J Biol Chem 266: 6365–6369
25. Martin DJ, Lluel P, Guillot E, Coste A, Jammes D, Angel I (1997) Comparative alpha-1 adrenoceptor subtype selectivity and functional uroselectivity of alpha-1 adrenoceptor antagonists. J Pharmacol Exp Ther 282: 228–235
26. Na YJ, Guo YL, Gu FL (1998) Clinical comparison of selective and non-selective alpha 1A-adrenoceptor antagonists for bladder outlet obstruction associated with benign prostatic hyperplasia: studies on tamsulosin and terazosin in Chinese patients. The Chinese Tamsulosin Study Group. J Med 29: 289–304
27. Neal DE (1994) Evaluation and results of treatments for prostatism [editorial]. Urol Res 22: 61–66
28. Neal DE, Ramsden PD, Sharples L, Smith A, Powell PH, Styles RA, Webb RJ (1989) Outcome of elective prostatectomy [see comments]. BMJ 299: 762–767
29. Perez DM, Piascik MT, Graham RM (1991) Solution-phase library screening for the identification of rare clones: isolation of an alpha 1D-adrenergic receptor cDNA. Mol Pharmacol 40: 876–883
30. Persson K, Sando JJ, Tuttle JB, Steers WD (1995) Protein kinase C in cyclic stretch-induced nerve growth factor production by urinary tract smooth muscle cells. Am J Physiol 269: C1018–C1024
31. Polder JJ, Meerding WJ, Koopmanschap MA, Bonneux L, van der Maas PJ (1994) The cost of disease in the Netherlands (in Dutch). Institute of Medical Technology Assessment

32. Ramarao CS, Denker JM, Perez DM, Gaivin RJ, Riek RP, Graham RM (1992) Genomic organization and expression of the human alpha 1B-adrenergic receptor. J Biol Chem 267: 21936–21945
33. Ruffolo RR Jr, Hieble JP (1999) Adrenoceptor pharmacology: urogenital applications. Eur Urol 36 [Suppl] 1: 17–22
34. Schwinn DA, Lomasney JW, Lorenz W, Szklut PJ, Fremeau RT Jr, Yang-Feng TL, Caron MG, Lefkowitz RJ, Cotecchia S (1990) Molecular cloning and expression of the cDNA for a novel alpha 1-adrenergic receptor subtype. J Biol Chem 265: 8183–8189
35. Scofield MA, Liu F, Abel PW, Jeffries WB (1995) Quantification of steady state expression of mRNA for alpha-1 adrenergic receptor subtypes using reverse transcription and a competitive polymerase chain reaction. J Pharmacol Exp Ther 275: 1035–1042
36. Seaman EK, Jacobs BZ, Blaivas JG, Kaplan SA (1994) Persistence or recurrence of symptoms after transurethral resection of the prostate: a urodynamic assessment. J Urol 152: 935–937
37. Starke K, Montel H, Gayk W, Merker R (1974) Comparison of the effects of clonidine on pre- and postsynaptic adrenoceptors in the rabbit pulmonary artery. Alpha-sympathomimetic inhibition of Neurogenic vasoconstriction. Naunyn Schmiedebergs Arch Pharmacol 285: 133–150
38. Steers WD, Albo M, Tuttle JB (1994) Calcium channel antagonists prevent urinary bladder growth and neuroplasticity following mechanical stress. Am J Physiol 266: R20–R26
39. Steers WD, Creedon DJ, Tuttle JB (1996) Immunity to nerve growth factor prevents afferent plasticity following urinary bladder hypertrophy. J Urol 155: 379–385
40. Uvelius B, Persson L, Mattiasson A (1984) Smooth muscle cell hypertrophy and hyperplasia in the rat detrusor after short-time infravesical outflow obstruction. J Urol 131: 173–176
41. Voigt MM, Kispert J, Chin HM (1990) Sequence of a rat brain cDNA encoding an alpha-1B adrenergic receptor. Nucleic Acids Res 18: 1053
42. Wein AJ, Levin RM (1979) Comparison of adrenergic receptor density in urinary bladder in man, dog, and rabbit. Surg Forum 30: 576–578
43. Wetzel JM, Miao SW, Forray C, Borden LA, Branchek TA, Gluchowski C (1995) Discovery of alpha 1a-adrenergic receptor antagonists based on the L-type Ca2+ channel antagonist niguldipine. J Med Chem 38: 1579–1581

Correspondence address: Christian Hampel, MD, Department of Urology, Johannes Gutenberg University Mainz, Langenbeckstrasse 1, D-55131 Mainz, Germany (E-mail: hampel@urologie.klinik.uni-mainz.de).

Calcium metabolism and detrusor failure in the aging bladder

D. Rohrmann

Department of Urology, University Hospital Aachen, Germany

Contents

1.   Physiology of bladder contraction

Bladder smooth muscle contraction depends on a transient rise in cytosolic free calcium that may be achieved by extracellular calcium influx through ion channels in the plasma membrane and by release from intracellular calcium storage sites. The neurotransmitter acetylcholine initiates excitation-contraction coupling. It binds to M3 receptors on the cell membrane and activates phospholipase C, an enzyme that induces the formation of inositol-1,4,5-triphosphate(IP3). IP3 is a second messenger that triggers the release of calcium from the intracellular storage sites. The existence of receptor operated intracellular calcium stores in the bladder was demonstrated by Mostwin (1985). They most likely comprise a heterogeneous group of organelles derived from the endoplasmic reticulum and may be referred to as sarcoplasmic reticulum (SR). A key component of the SR is an energy dependent calcium pump, which serves to drive free calcium out of the cytosol back into the storage sites. It was first described by Maclennan (1970) and is called sarcoplasmic endoplasmic reticulum calcium-magnesium-adenosinetriphosphatase (SERCA). SERCA is located on the surface of the SR and it pumps 1 free calcium ion into the SR per molecule of adenosine triphosphate consumed.

2.   Bladder outlet obstruction

In animal models of bladder outlet obstruction, the increase of bladder outlet resistance results in a variety of changes. Results can be contradictory depending on the animal model used and the degree of obstruction. Mild obstruction may lead to bladder hyperactivity while severe and long-lasting obstruction usually results in detrusor function failure. In some cases after a period of partial compensation a bladder with long-term obstruction will have delayed decompensation. The molecular basis for the mechanisms of compensation and decompensation is quite unclear. It is a complex process that reflects changes in many pathways one of which is intracellular calcium metabolism.

2.1   Animal model

All studies were done using mature male New Zealand white rabbits. The urethra was intubated with an 8F catheter and exposed through a lower midline incision. A 4-0 silk suture was passed around the proximal urethra and tied over the catheter.

At the desired experimental time points (7, 14 and 28 days) the bladders were removed and the detrusor muscle was investigated as described below.

2.2   Smooth muscle physiology

Smooth muscle strips (1 mm × 1 mm × 10 mm) from the detrusor were mounted in an organ bath that contained Tyrode's solution (125 mmol sodium chloride, 2.7 mmol potassium chloride, 0.4 mmol sodium phosphate, 0.5 mmol magnesium chloride, 23.8 mmol sodium bicarbonate and 1% glucose) and was supplied with 95% oxygen and 5% carbon dioxide. After equilibration for 1 hour at slack length strips were stretched in increments of 2.5 mm. After waiting 10 minutes field stimulation (32 Hz, 80V) was applied and active tension was measured. L_0 was defined as the length where maximal force was generated. Peak tension was measured in response to field stimulation and 200 µM Bethanechol. All strips were weighed at completion of the experiments. The results recorded from the polygraph were corrected for strip weight and expressed as gm tension per 100 mg tissue.

2.3   Biochemical assay for SERCA activity

Thapsigargin is a substance that selectively inhibits SERCA activity. It was used to develop the assay described below (Zderic et al. 1996).

1 gm of thawed tissue was processed in a special fashion combining several steps of centrifugation to isolate microsomal membranes. 100 µl of membranes were used for each assay. 0.2 cc of 40 mM adenosine triphosphate, 0.2 cc of 40 mM calcium chloride and 1.5 cc TRIS-hydrochloride buffer were added. Phosphate release was then determined by withdrawing aliquots of 0.334 cc at 0, 10, 20, 30 and 40 minutes of elapsed time. The adenosinetriphosphatase reaction in the aliquots was quenched by 0.166 cc 12.5% trichloroacetic acid. To this was then added 1 cc distilled water and

0.5 cc ferrous sulfate-ammonium-molybdate reagent. The solution was thoroughly vortexed and after 5 minutes optical density at 650 nm was measured. The basis of phosphate determination was the colorimetric measurement of the phosphate molybdate complex.

To determine adenosinetriphosphatase activity due to SERCA the inhibitor thapsigargin was added to a second assay done in parallel on the identical membrane preparation. The activity attributable to SERCA was defined as total adenosinetriphosphatase activity minus that in the presence of thapsigargin. Statistical comparison was done using the Student's t test with significance at $p < 0.05$.

2.4   Western blot

To corroborate our results, we used immunoblotting after gel electrophoretic separation of the membrane proteins. The monoclonal antibody used was specific for SERCA. The membrane fraction samples were dissolved in 6% sodium dodecyl sulfate buffer containing 50 mM dithiothreitol, 10 mM ethylenediaminetetraacetic acid, 100 μg/cc benzamidine, 40 μg/cc phenyl-methylsulfonylfluoride, 1 mM iodoacetamine, 500 mM sucrose and 130 mM TRIS-hydrochloride. After 20 minutes at 4C and 3 minutes at 100C standard gel electrophoresis was done.

Proteins from the gel were blotted onto a nitrocellulose membrane using an electroblot transfer. The membrane was immersed in 5% nonfat dry milk in 5% phosphate buffered saline for 1 hour, then the SERCA antibody was added and incubated with the membrane overnight at 4C. After careful rinsing with PBS-buffer incubation with an antimouse immunoglobin G conjugated with horseradish peroxidase antibody for a 2-hour period at room temperature was done. Color was developed by adding a solution of 5 cc chloronaphthol. The solutions were developed at room temperature with shaking until bands appeared.

3.   The effects of bladder outlet obstruction on SERCA activity

Bladder outlet obstruction resulted in a decrease of contractility. The degree of functional impairment was paralleled by an increase in bladder weight and not dependent on the duration of obstruction (Table 1)

The evaluation of SERCA activity confirmed a very good correlation to functional impairment (Fig. 1) For SERCA all values were statistically significant versus control tissue. We found that each bladder reacts different to bladder outlet obstruction and this is probably due to the degree of obstruction in each experimental setup. We therefore elected to group the bladders according to their functional properties into two groups: compensated and decompensated bladders. We defined bladders as compensated when the force generated by the muscle strips exceeded 50% of control group forces. Decompensated was defined as bladder smooth muscle strips

Table 1. Experimental results for each time point of obstruction

	Control	No. wks.		
		1	2	4
Bladder wt. (gm.)	1.9 ± 0.1	$9.9 \pm 2.1^{\dagger}$	$5.4 \pm 1.3^{*}$	$8.3 \pm 2.3^{*}$
Bethanechol (200 μM.)	20.3 ± 2.1	$5.3 \pm 1.0^{*}$	13.7 ± 3.0	$5.4 \pm 1.3^{*}$
Field stimulation (volts)	11 ± 3.2	$1.6 \pm 0.3^{*}$	15.9 ± 4.0	$8.8 \pm 5^{*}$
Protein/wet wt. (mg./gm.)	1.3 ± 0.1	1.4 ± 0.1	$2.1 \pm 0.3^{*}$	$2.6 \pm 0.3^{*}$
SERCA:				
Nmol./min./mg. protein	366 ± 9	$83 \pm 13^{\dagger}$	$187 \pm 50^{*}$	$128 \pm 33^{\dagger}$
Nmol./min./gm. wet wt.	281 ± 7	$59 \pm 10^{\dagger}$	$89 \pm 23^{\dagger}$	$50 \pm 13^{\dagger}$
SERCA/total adenosinetriphosphatase (%)	25 ± 3	$19 \pm 3^{*}$	$17 \pm 3^{*}$	$15 \pm 4^{*}$

Values are expressed as means plus or minus standard error of mean
* $p < 0.05$
† $p < 0.01$

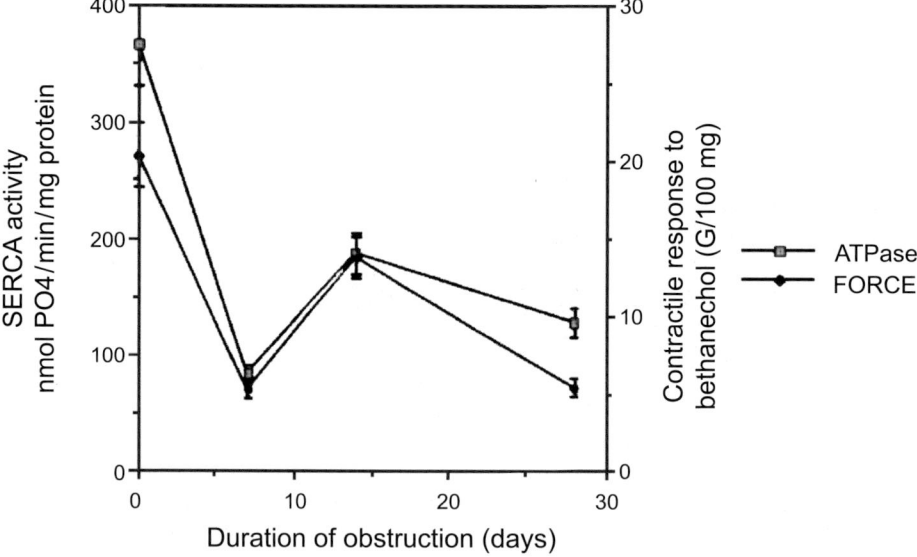

Fig. 1. Relationship between contractile force generation and SERCA activity as function of duration of obstruction

in which the force generated was less than 50% of control. Using this method of analysis we defined three major classes: control, compensated and decompensated. Table 2 shows the average data for these groups. There are significant differences in bladder weight, response to electrical field stimulation and to bethanechol stimulation. SERCA activity is expressed in Fig. 2. Interestingly, the proportion of adenosinetriphosphatase activity

Table 2. Experimental data stratified according to functional performance

	Control	Compensated	Decompensated
Bladder wt. (gm.)	1.9 ± 0.1	$3.6 \pm 0.7^*$	$9.9 \pm 1.4^†$
Bethanechol (200 µM.)	20.3 ± 2.8	$18.7 \pm 1.7^*$	$5.5 \pm 0.7^†$
Field stimulation (volts)	11 ± 3.2	18.8 ± 3	$2.1 \pm 0.5^†$
Protein/wet wt. (mg./gm.)	1.3 ± 0.1	1.8 ± 0.2	2.0 ± 0.2
SERCA:			
Nmol./min./mg. protein	366 ± 16	$233 \pm 31^*$	$83 \pm 11^†$
Nmol./min./gm. wet wt.	279 ± 11	$131 \pm 12^*$	$41 \pm 6^†$
SERCA/total adenosinetriphosphatase (%)	25 ± 3	$16 \pm 2^*$	$18 \pm 2^*$

Values are expressed as means plus or minus standard error of mean
$^*\, p < 0.05$ versus control
$^†\, p < 0.01$ versus control

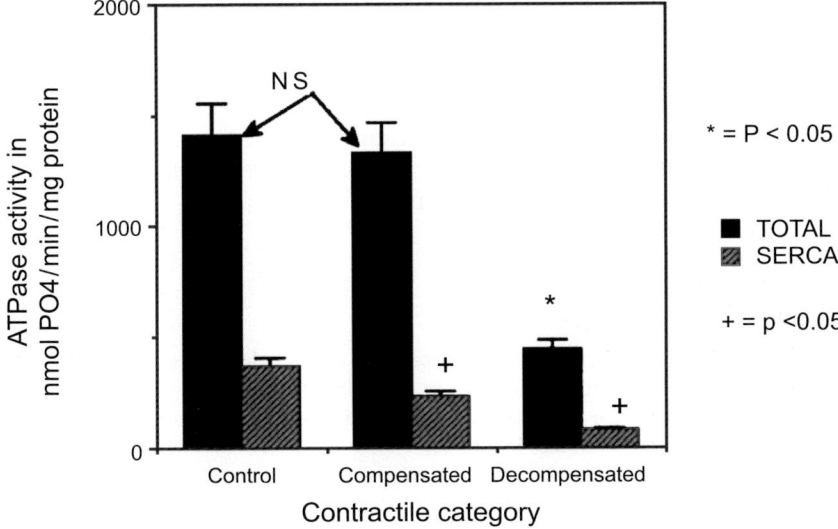

Fig. 2. Relationship between total adenosinetriphosphatase (ATPase) activity and SERCA specific activity for groups depending on contractile status (compensated or decompensated)

accounted for by SERCA already decreases in the compensated group while the total adenosinetriphosphatase activity remains unchanged compared to controls. This suggests SERCA activity to be a very sensitive marker for functional impairment.

Figure 3 shows the Western blots. The expression of SERCA immunoreactivity was greatest in the control bladder. In the obstructed group there was some loss of signal intensity. However, in the group deemed to be decompensated there was virtually no detectable immunoreactivity.

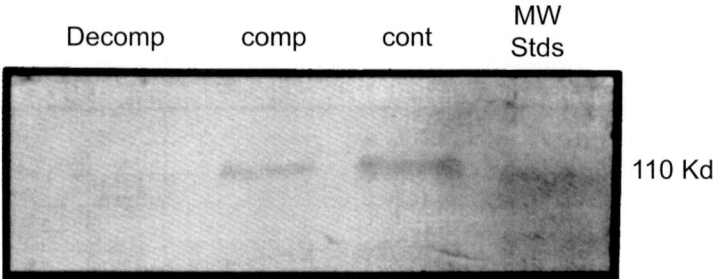

Fig. 3. Western blot form control (Cont), compensated (Comp) and decompensated (Decomp) bladder smooth muscle

4. Closing remarks

The role of intracellular calcium stores in bladder smooth muscle was evaluated in an animal experimental setup. We found that the activity of SERCA, the sarcoplasmic endoplasmic reticulum calcium-magnesium-adenosintriphosphatase, correlates well with functional impairment after bladder outlet obstruction. SERCA serves to drive free calcium ions out of the cytosol back into the storage sites. Even in bladders with preserved function the activity of SERCA is already markedly decreased.

We speculate that SERCA is an early marker of impending functional impairment in the presence of bladder outlet obstruction.

5. References

1. Maclennan D (1970) Purification and properties of an adenosinetriphosphatase from sarcoplasmic retriculum. J Biol Chem 245: 4508
2. Mostwin JL (1985) Receptor operated intracellular calcium stores in the smooth muscle of the guinea pig bladder. J Urol 133: 900
3. Zderic SA, Rohrmann D, Gong C, Snyder HM, Duckett JW, Wein AJ, Levin RM (1996) The decompsated detrusor II. Evidence of loss of sarcomplasic reticulum function following bladder outlet obstruction in the rabbit. J Urol 156: 587–592

Correspondence address: Dorothea Rohrmann M.D., Universitätsklinikum Aachen, Pauwelsstrasse 30, D-52057 Aachen, Germany (E-mail: drohrmann@ukaachen.de).

The significance of the urine-blood-barrier for urge generation and possible changes in the aging bladder

C. R. Riedl

Department of Urology, Thermenklinikum Baden, Baden, Austria

Contents

1.   The aging bladder – an *urgent* problem

As a real challenge in current practice, urologists see a growing number of patients with age-related bladder symptoms. In a recent survey we found a 12.5% rate of functional bladder disorders among urology patients in the age group of 60–80, that increased to 34.5% for patients >80 years (Daha et al. 2002). But the frequency and importance of these problems is not yet reflected by an adequate number of research projects and publications. Only 3‰ of presentations throughout the last annual meetings of the American Urological Association (AUA) covered the topic of age-related changes to urological organ systems, with only a minimal share regarding the urinary bladder.

At least, three important statements on age-related changes to the bladder and micturition have been made.

1. The circadian rhythm of diuresis shows an increase of nocturnal diuresis in older patients. This may be consequent to hormonal or cardiovascular changes. The conclusion is that nocturia is a natural event in older people and less relevant as a symptom (Morgan et al. 2000).
2. Moderate detrusor ischemia may lead to detrusor hyperreflexia, and severe ischemia to detrusor fibrosis with hypercontractility (Azadzoi et al. 1999).
3. The basal release of acetylcholine, the main neurotransmitter in bladder contraction, is increased in older people and may contribute to age-related changes in bladder function and hyperreflexia (Yoshida et al. 2002).

Nocturia, better nocturnal polyuria, as well as detrusor hyperreflexia are the main urological symptoms affecting aging people. Various therapeutic regimens are available for the treatment of obstructive voiding disorders and incontinence but, in contrast to that, urgency and frequency are still a problem for patients and doctors, since common treatments are ineffective in a high proportion of cases. In the presence of global mobility, uncontrolled urgency and reduced functional bladder capacity result in the impossibility of leaving the home area and are extremely disabling and distressing to patients.

2.   The physiology of urge generation and control

The base for treating age related urgency efficiently is a correct understanding of the physiological processes responsible for urge generation that are essentially related to the urine-blood-barrier (Hohlbrugger and Riedl 2000). While recent concepts favour a neuromechanical model for urge induction with mechanoreceptors stimulated by bladder distension, older concepts also included chemoceptive stimulation of the suburothelial C-fibres as responsible for urge sensation. Urgency in case of acute cystitis consequent to increased urothelial permeability as an inflammatory reaction is an excellent example for chemically induced C-fibre stimulation.

The present understanding of urge generation has to include both chemoceptive and neuromechanical concepts. The sensitive region for chemoception is the urine-blood-barrier, which morphologically consists of the urothelium (generally permeable for urinary compounds) and glycosaminoglycanes (GAG-layer). Glycosaminoglycanes are mucopolysaccharides consisting of hyaluronic acid, heparin, chondroitin sulfate, and dermatan sulfate (Parsons et al. 1990).

The high gradient of urinary compounds between urine, the suburothelial tissue, and blood (1:10 for potassium, 1:4.5 for urea) is a great challenge for this barrier. Maintenance of these gradients is of vital importance for body homeostasis and prevents recirculation of substances excreted by the kidneys. Very efficiently, a suburothelial microvascular countercurrent system (Fig. 1), similar to the one in the tubular system of the kidney, prevents penetration of transurothelially diffused urinary compounds, especially potassium, to deeper layers of the bladder wall. If potassium reached the detrusor this would result in immediate depolarisation and contraction of the detrusor smooth muscle cells. Via veno-arterial shunting the resorbed components of the urine recirculate in exchange for plasma water, and are thus diluted in the venous blood and retained in the suburothelial region (Steers 1998, Hohlbrugger 1995, Miodonski and Litwin 1999, Rosamilia et al. 1999). This effective vascular system is responsible for keeping potassium and hydrogen ions away from the chemoceptive suburothelial C-fibre endings. Under normal circumstances, the chemoceptive excitation of the C-fibres from potassium or hydrogen ions does not cross the threshold of the cerebral cortex as long as the integrity of the

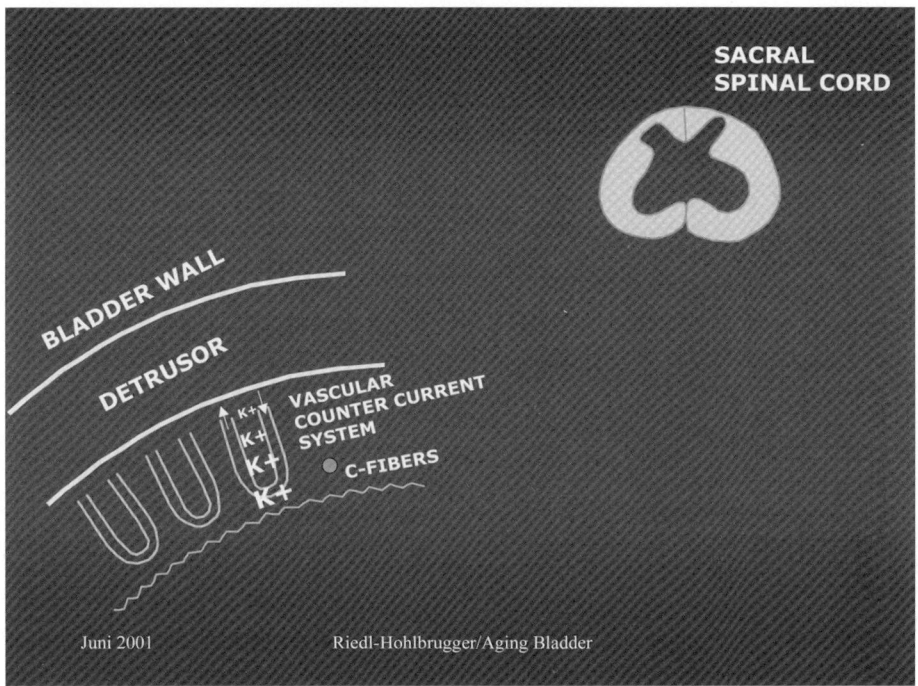

Fig. 1. Suburothelial vascular counter current system protects detrusor from potassium overflow

entire urothelium is maintained. However, in case of increased urothelial permeability, such as during acute inflammation or chronic interstitial cystitis, the suburothelial space is flooded by urinary compounds that cannot sufficiently be washed out by the suburothelial vascular plexus. In turn, C-fibres are stimulated to an extent that neuronal excitation is propagated to the sacral micturition centre. Consequently, via afferent cholinergic fibres, stimulation of detrusor muscle cells is effected (Morrison et al. 1999).

The detrusor muscle is a smooth muscle with an unstable membrane potential (similar to all other hollow organs) that is destabilized mechanically by increasing distension (bladder filling), as well as chemically by potassium ions and low pH via C-fibre induced cholinergic activity from the sacral micturition centre.

The activation status of the detrusor muscle membrane potential is "recorded" by A-δ-fibres and "reported" to the sacral as well as the pontine micturition centre, with the final sensation of urge generated in the cortex (Heng et al. 1999, van Asselt et al. 1999). The pontine micturition centre downregulates urgency via the adrenergic system that directly inhibits A-δ-activity (Fig. 2). As a second mechanism for urge reduction, an adrenergic increase of suburothelial blood flow is induced to maintain the concentration gradients of urinary compounds within the bladder wall and to wash out potassium and hydrogen ions by an increase of plasma filtration.

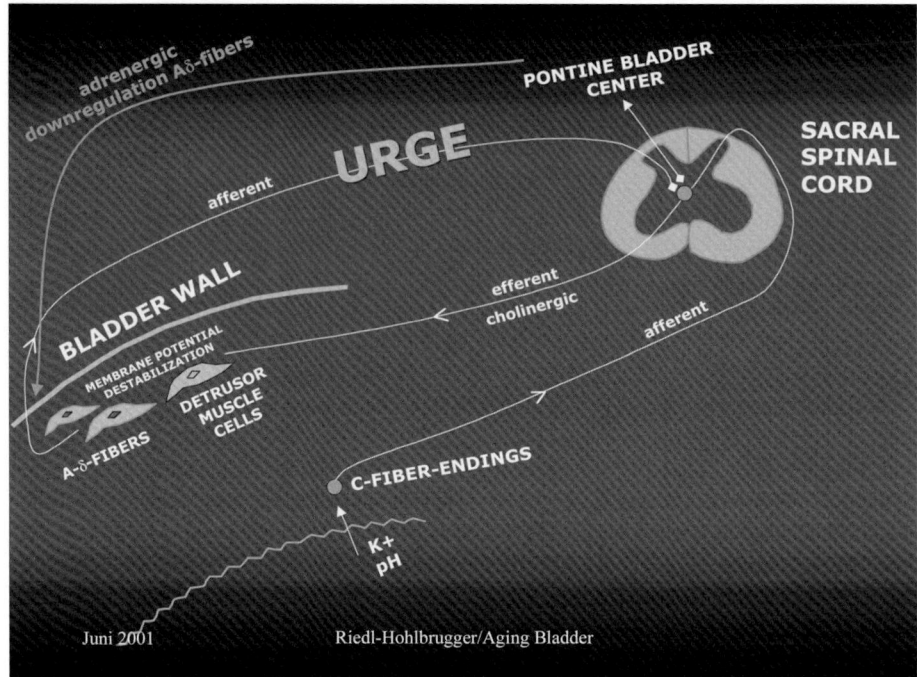

Fig. 2. Urge generation and its control by adrenergic mechanisms

This filling- and medium-dependent increase of bladder wall perfusion has been shown by Hohlbrugger (Hohlbrugger et al. 2000): potassium chloride instillation leads to a higher rate of blood flow compared with instillation of saline, as to prevent an inadequate sensation of urgency provoked by the high potassium concentration.

A successful control of urinary urge presupposes normal function of the cortex over the pontine continence centre. Otherwise, as soon as a specific afferent excitation threshold is exceeded, the continence centre is automatically switched off and the topographically neighbouring micturition centre switched on (as found in children before they reach the age of bladder control) (Blok and Holstege 1999). The impulse from the continence centre is exclusively directed along the sympathetic innervation of the bladder and the sympatho-somatic innervation of the sphincter apparatus. Consequently, as mentioned before, these adrenergic impulses, (1) reduce detrusor activity (counterbalancing the cholinergic C-fibre-mediated input), and (2) increase the vesical blood flow as well as (3) the smooth and striated sphincter tonicity.

In summary, generation of urge is as complex as its control, and a multitude of physiologic mechanisms are necessary to secure adequate excretion of renal waste in a controllable way. With special regard to the blood-urine-barrier, i.e. the bladder wall with its high concentration gradients, the understanding of these physiological processes of urge generation and urge control results in five key points for possible age-related changes of this system. Besides overt causes as infections, malignancies or urinary stones, there are several reasons for increased urgency.

3.   Causes of increased urgency

May be consequent to:

1. Urothelial damage with primary or secondary deficiency of the GAG-layer, resulting in an increased urothelial permeability with increased potassium penetration and urge sensation at inadequate low bladder filling volumes (easily demonstrable with the modified potassium chloride test as introduced later).
2. Vascular deficiency (general/regional perfusion disorders) with a decrease of suburothelial perfusion and a deficit in potassium washout. As mentioned before, there is proof that chronic ischaemia not only induces morphological changes of the urothelium and the detrusor, but also provokes instable detrusor contractions. The animal model introduced by Adzadzoi seems to be excellently suited for examining whether ischaemia increases or reduces permeability or susceptibility of the urothelium to inflammation other than that caused by infection (Azadzoi et al. 1999).
3. General adrenergic hypoactivity, most probably drug-induced (α- and β-blocking drugs are commonly prescribed for cardiovascular reasons in a high proportion of older people), resulting in a deficient central urge down-regulation at the level of the A-δ-fibres as well as in the impossibility of inducing an increase of suburothelial perfusion.
4. Muscular deficiency, possibly of degenerative origin, with primary or secondary destabilization of the detrusor membrane potential. This may be the consequence of various diseases, mainly metabolic (diabetes mellitus, etc.) or toxic (drug or alcohol abuse, environmental, etc.).
5. Neurological disorders with an impaired regulation of afferent, efferent, peripheral, or central parts of the complex urge regulation system. This group comprises cortical deficiencies (stroke, tumours, etc.) as well as neuropathic diseases of multiple origin (diabetes, toxic, etc.)

4.   Is urgency similar in the aging bladder and in interstitial cystitis?

Our longstanding experience with interstitial cystitis (IC), the chronic disease resulting from increased urothelial permeability, established one hypothesis for age-related urgency: the possible damage to the blood-urine barrier (with the cascade of urinary overflow of the suburothelial space that cannot be washed out and compensated by increased suburothelial blood flow, K^+- and H^+-triggered excitation of the C-fibres and, finally, the cholinergically destabilised detrusor muscle) (Hohlbrugger 1996, Parsons et al. 1991, Parsons et al. 1998, Teichman and Nielsen-Omeis 1999).

The potassium sensitivity in patients with increased urothelial permeability can be demonstrated easily: Parsons introduced a specific test by simply instilling 0.4 M KCl in the bladders of IC patients (Parsons 1999). This test qualitatively evaluates the urothelial permeability status, however, it is extremely painful for most IC patients. Thus, it cannot be recommended for routine use. The modified potassium test with 0.2 M KCl as introduced by Hohlbrugger is better tolerated and should be considered the current state of the art examination for diagnosis of early stage IC (Hohlbrugger 1999).

No more is needed than two solutions for instillation (0.9% sodium chloride and 0.2 M KCl), an infusion set, a catheter, and a measuring cup. Maximal bladder capacity is first determined with saline and then with the 0.2 M KCl solution. A >30% reduction of maximal bladder capacity with 0.2 M KCl filling compared to saline is considered evidence of increased urothelial permeability.

In a study performed at our institution, the modified potassium test with comparative assessment of maximal bladder capacity (Cmax) was performed in 40 patients with IC and 38 controls (Daha et al. 2002). Controls did not show a significant difference in Cmax with either solution. KCl reduced Cmax in 37/40 (92%) IC patients with a mean Cmax reduction of 30%. The examination was painless in all controls and in 33/40 (82%) IC patients and was moderately painful in 7 IC patients. The three patients with no reduction of Cmax on 0.2 M KCl were all reactive when 0.4 M KCl was instilled. In summary, comparative assessment of Cmax is a well tolerated alternative to the original 0.4 M test for diagnosis of increased urothelial permeability/IC, sparing most patients the pain of higher potassium concentrations. In addition, the modified version is a quantitative evaluation compared to the original test, which simplifies comparison of inter- and intraindividual results.

In our experience, a positive potassium sensitivity test is only observed in about 10% of patients with urgency as an aging bladder symptom. There is a clear difference between both patients groups: IC patients suffer from an enhanced urothelial permeability that generates sensory urgency via the C-fibres as well as direct detrusor depolarisation (=hypocontractility), whereas aging bladder patients present with motoric urgency due to uninhibited detrusor hyperactivity. However, it is important to detect this low number of IC patients among the group of aging bladder patients, since they are mostly cured with GAG substitution therapy that restores the normal urine-tissue barrier. According to our personal experience, a success rate of up to 85% can be expected in patients with interstitial cystitis if treatment is initiated at an early stage.

5.   Glycosaminogylcane-substitution/instillation therapy

Today several drugs are available for instillation therapy: hyaluronic acid, pentosanpolysulphate (PPS, a semi-synthetic heparin analog), and heparin.

Apart from restoring the GAG layer several further therapeutic mechanisms are postulated for these drugs:

- Reduction of leukocytic and immunological effects inside the bladder wall
- Thus, reduction of inflammatory reactions
- Regulation and improvement of connective tissue regeneration
- Restoration of the suburothelial barrier of the lamina propria
- Neutralization of oxygen radicals in the bladder wall

With hyaluronic acid, a single instillation of 40 mg per week is sufficient to achieve the desired therapeutic effect. In most cases 10–12 instillations are performed, followed by a gradual reduction to one instillation per month (Morales et al. 1996).

A similar efficacy has been observed for instillation treatment with PPS, usually at a dosage of 300 mg three times a week for a period of at least three months (Bade et al. 1997, Hwang et al. 1997, Nickel et al. 2002). PPS is the only drug that is also available in an oral formulation. In contrast, heparin seems to be less effective as single therapy, but may be used in combination with either hyaluronic acid or PPS (Parsons et al. 1994).

In the past, DMSO (dimethylsulfoxid) was often used as an inexpensive instillation treatment. However, this treatment will not restore the GAG-layer; in contrast, the effect is partial destruction of the urothelium followed by recovery of a competent urothelium and GAG production. Currently, DMSO therapy can no longer be recommended, as it is associated with various inconvenient side effects (post-instillation pain, garlic odour) and less effective than other drugs.

The principal therapeutic measures in IC besides instillation therapy that may also be used for treatment of urge symptoms in the aging bladder can be categorised as follows:

- Elimination of etiologic agents (coffeine, cold, drugs, provoking food, excitement/stress)
- Additional drug therapy
- Additional physiotherapeutic and psychotherapeutic treatment (Pudendus nerve stimulation, magnetic field therapy, bladder training) (Primus and Kramer 1996).

6.   New perspectives

Additional oral drugs that are effective in IC patients may be beneficial for the aging bladder syndrome, too. Cranberry juice, an old Indian medicine against "bladder problems," contains anthocyanes, which reduce the patient's susceptibility to urinary tract infections by reducing bacterial adhesion to the urothelium and probably restoring the urine-tissue barrier similar to GAG's (Howell et al. 1998). In single studies, the tricyclic antidepressant amitriptyline effectively reduced symptoms of interstitial cystitis (Sant 1997). In our experience, it is a valuable additive in patients suffering from urgency of any cause.

Future therapeutic perspectives are mainly directed to new detrusor inactivating drugs, since cholinergics are only effective to a limited extent. Botulinum toxin may be used to selectively eliminate parts of the detrusor muscle and thus reduce contractility (Smith et al. 2002, Chancellor and Smith 2002). Preliminary observations suggest that vanillinoids (capsaicin, resiniferatoxin), in spite of their ability to reduce C-fibre activity, are less likely to increase the reduced functional capacity of the aging bladder (de Seze et al. 1999). Sacral neuromodulation may effectively resolve urgency in at least part of the patients (Wyndaele et al. 2000, Schmidt et al. 1999).

7.   Conclusion

Common morbidity is increased with age, and a multitude of causes, alone or in combination, may be responsible for one of the five mechanisms possibly inducing urgency in the aging bladder. Age-related changes, in the normal physiological as well as in the pathological range, result in perfusion disorders, neuropathies, metabolic disorders, and apoptotic cell reduction. Last but not least, numerous drugs may influence the complex urge regulation system. As it seems, the aging bladder is not a single disorder of a single organ, but the result of multiple, possibly minimal, changes of various organ systems. Future studies have to evaluate the significance of each of these hypothetic causes for the aging bladder syndrome. Only identification of the pathogenetic mechanisms responsible for the aging bladder syndrome will help us find effective therapeutic regimens to spare old people the experience of a life dominated by the functionality or dysfunctionality of their bladder.

8.   References

1. Azadzoi KM, Tarcan T, Kozlowski R, Krane RJ, Siroky MB (1999) Overactivity and structural changes in the chronically ischemic bladder. J Urol 162: 1768–1778
2. Azazdoi KM, Tarcan T, Siroky MB, Krane RJ (1999) Atherosclerosis-induced chronic ischaemia causes bladder fibrosis and non-compliance in the rabbit. J Urol 161: 1626–1635
3. Bade JJ, Laseur M, Nieuwenburg A, van der Weele LT, Mensink HJ (1997) A placebo-controlled study of intravesical pentosanpolysulphate for the treatment of interstitial cystitis. BJU Int 79: 168–171
4. Blok BF, Holstege G (1999) The central control of micturition and continence: implications for urology. BJU Int 83 [Suppl]: 1–6
5. Chancellor M, Smith CP (2002) One surgeon's experience in 50 patients with botulinum toxin injection into the bladder and urethra. J Urol 167 [Suppl]: 981A
6. Daha LK, Riedl CR, Hohlbrugger G, Knoll M, Engelhardt PF, Pflüger H (2003) Comparative assessment of maximal bladder capacity, 0.9% NaCl vs. 0.2 M KCl, for the diagnosis of interstitial cystitis: a prospective controlled study. J Urol (in press)

7. Daha KL, Riedl CR, Simak R, Engelhardt PF, Plas E, Pflüger H (2002) Incidence of urologic diseases in geriatric patients in a large community hospital. J Am Ger Soc 50(9): 159–160

8. de Seze M, Wiart L, Ferriere J, de Seze MP, Joseph P, Barat M (1999) Intravesical instillation of capsaicin in urology: A review of the literature. Eur Urol 36: 267–277

9. Heng CL, Liu JC, Chang SY (1999) Effect of capsaicin on the micturition reflex in normal and chronic spinal cord-injured cats. Am J Physiol 277: R786–R794

10. Hohlbrugger G (1995) The vesical blood-urine barrier: a relevant and dynamic interface between renal function and nervous bladder control. J Urol 154: 6–15

11. Hohlbrugger G (1996) Leaky urothelium and/or vesical ischaemia enable urinary potassium to cause idiopathic urgency/frequency syndrome and urge incontinence. Int Urogynecol J Pelvic Floor Dysfunction 7: 242–255

12. Hohlbrugger G (1999) Urinary potassium and the overactive bladder. BJU Int 83 [Suppl 2]: 22–28

13. Hohlbrugger G, Frauscher F, Strasser H, Stenzl A, Bartsch G (2000) Evidence for autoregulation of vesical circulation by intravesical potassium chloride and distension in the normal human bladder. BJU Int 85: 412–415

14. Hohlbrugger G, Riedl CR (2000) Non-bacterial cystitis. Curr Opinion Urol 10: 371–380

15. Howell AB, Vorsa N, der Marderosian A, Foo L (1998) Inhibition of the adherence of E.Coli to uroepithelial surfaces by poranthocyandin extracts from cranberries. NEJM 339: 1085–1086

16. Hwang P, Auclair B, Beechinor D, Diment M, Einarson TR (1997) Efficacy of pentosan polysulfate in the treatment of interstitial cystitis: a meta-analysis. Urology 50: 39–43

17. Interstitial Cystitis (1994) Urol Clinics North Am 21, 2

18. Interstitial Cystitis (1997) An update of current information. Urology 49: 5A

19. Miodonski AJ, Litwin JA (1999) Microvascular architecture of the human urinary bladder wall: a corosion casting study. Anat Rec 254: 375–381

20. Morales A, Emerson L, Nickel JC, Lundie M (1996) Intravesical hyaluronic acid in the treatment of refractory interstitial cystitis. J Urol 156: 45–48

21. Morgan KA, Bergmann MA, Kiely DK (2000) The voiding pattern of normal elders. J Urol 163 [Suppl]: 1012A

22. Morrison J, Wen J, Kibble A (1999) Activation of pelvic afferent nerves from the rat bladder during filling. Scand J Urol Nephrol 201 [Suppl]: 73–75

23. Nickel CJ, Forrest J, Tomera KM (2002) Effects of pentosan polysulfate sodium in men with chronic pelvic pain syndrome: a multicenter randomized placebo-controlled study. J Urol 167 [Suppl]: 248A

24. Parsons CL (1999) Potassium sensitivity test. Techniques in Urology 2: 171–173

25. Parsons CL, Boychuk D, Jones S, Hurst R, Callahan H (1990) Bladder surface glycosaminoglykanes: an epithelial permeability barrier. J Urol 143: 139–142

26. Parsons CL, Greenberger M, Gabal L, Bidair M, Barme G (1998) The role of urinary potassium in the pathogenesis and diagnosis of interstitial cystitis. J Urol 159: 1862–1867

27. Parsons CL, Housley T, Schmidt JD, Lebow D (1994) Treatment of interstitial cystitis with intravesical heparin. BJU 73: 504–507

28. Parsons CL, Lilly JD, Stein P (1991) Epithelial dysfunction in nonbacterial cystitis (Interstitial Cystitis). J Urol 145: 732–735

29. Primus G, Kramer G (1996) Maximal external electrical stimulation for treatment of neurogenic or non-neurogenic urgency and/or urge incontinence. Neurourol Urodyn 15: 187–194
30. Rosamilia A, Clements JA, Dwyer PL, Kende M, Campbell DJ (1999) Bladder microvasculature in women with interstitial cystitis. J Urol 162: 330–334
31. Sant GR (1997) Interstitial Cystitis. Lippincott-Raven: Philadelphia, New York
32. Schmidt RA, Jonas U, Oleson KA, Janknegt RA, Hassouna MM, Siegel SW, van Kerrebroeck PE (1999) Sacral nerve stimulation for treatment of refractory urinary urge incontinence. Sacral Nerve Stimulation Study Group. J Urol 162: 352–357
33. Smith CP, Fraser MO, Bartho L (2002) Botulinum toxin A inhibits afferent nerve evoked bladder strip contractions. J Urol 167 [Suppl]: 164A
34. Steers WD (1998) Physiology and pharmacology of the bladder and urethra. In: Walsh PC, Retik AB, Vaughan ED Jr, Wein AJ (eds) Campbell's urology, 1, 7th edn. W.B. Saunders Company: Philadelphia, pp 870–915
35. Teichman JM, Nielsen-Omeis BJ (1999) Potassium leak test predicts outcome in interstitial cystitis. J Urol 161: 1791–1794
36. van Asselt E, le Feber J, van Mastrigt R (1999) Threshold for efferent bladder nerve firing in the rat. Am J Physiol 276: R1819–R1824
37. Wyndaele JJ, Michielsen D, van Dromme S (2000) Influence of sacral neuro-modulation on electrosensation of the lower urinary tract. J Urol 163: 221–224
38. Yoshida M, Inadome A, Murakami S (2002) Effects of age and muscle stretching on acetylcholine release in isolated human bladder smooth muscles. J Urol 167 [Suppl]: 160A

Correspondence address: Claus Riedl, MD, Department of Urology, Thermen-klinikum Baden, Wimmergasse 19, A-2500 Baden, Austria (E-Mail: claus.riedl@thermenklinikum-baden.at).

The impact of changes in fluid regulation hormones during aging

J. C. Djurhuus and *G. M. Hvistendahl*

International Enuresis Research Center,
Institute of Experimental Clinical Research,
Skejby Hospital, Aarhus, Denmark

Contents

1.   Introduction

Biological aging occurs on many different levels from the molecular level, through cells and organs, to the entire body and mind. The individual and the different organs and organ systems age at different rates. As a result, old people often differ more from one another than young people.

In practice it is difficult to distinguish aging and age related changes, endogenous and exogenous changes. As far as the urinary system is concerned it is evident that biological aging do occur but the impact of the changes on the related organs remains debatable (Hald and Horn 1998).

Elderly people experience all kinds of symptoms from the urinary tract more often than young people. Symptoms such as frequency, urgency, incontinence, and nocturia are often reported from elderly people. The origin of the underlying changes leading to these symptoms may derive from any level in the urinary tract, since changes in one organ may lead to changes in related organs. To be able to understand the mechanisms behind aging and symptoms caused by aging in the urinary tract system, it is necessary to study the inter-organic relation. A lot of anatomical and functional changes occur with aging, and these changes may influence the capacity of the bladder and the urine production in the kidneys.

1.1   The kidneys

With age total kidney mass decreases. The kidney volume is changing by 20–30%. Furthermore the renal blood flow decreases; cortical blood flow decreases more than medullary flow does. The response to vasodilators is reduced, as is the glomerular filtration rate. Also the conservation and excretion of sodium are impaired, leading to changes in the concentration and dilution of the urine. These changes are least in healthy individuals and most marked in those with coexisting morbidity, particularly cardiovascular disease (Rodger 1998). Clearly these changes above the bladder level will affect bladder function.

1.2   The bladder and urethra

It is evident that aging causes increased lower urinary tract symptoms (LUTS) owing to a decline in bladder capacity, detrusor contractility, and the ability to withhold voiding. The maximal urethral closure pressure and length probably decline in women, and detrusor overactivity increases in prevalence. The post-void residual probably increases to 50–100 ml (Diokno et al. 1988, Resnick 1988, Resnick 1990, Resnick et al. 1995). The prostate enlarges with age in most men, causing urodynamic bladder-outlet obstruction (BOO) in about half (Resnick et al. 1995). It is difficult to separate the effects of BOO from those related to aging. Furthermore LUTS is complicated by conditions that may affect the urinary bladder – for example, degenerative (multiple sclerosis), metabolic (diabetes mellitus), or neurogenic diseases. These diseases may be age-related either because the incidence increases with age, or, with chronic disease, the incidence of complications increases with duration of the disease and thus the increasing age.

1.3   Changes in fluid metabolism

In healthy young adults aged 21–35 the nocturnal urine production is approximately 14% of the total 24-hour urine production (Robertson et al. 1999), whereas people over the age of 65 have to excrete on average 34% of the urine production during night (Rembratt et al. 2000) (Kirkland et al. 1983). The day/night ratio of 24-hour urine production in elderly persons varies in different studies from 0.7 to 1.5 (Asplund and Aberg 1992, Carter et al. 1999) (Kirkland et al. 1983), and in younger people the ratio is 2.7 (Rittig et al. 1989). This illustrates a tremendous physiological change in the fluid metabolism. Therefore nocturia based on a changed fluid regulation becomes a very common symptom in the elderly population.

2.   Definition of nocturia

Nocturia is considered as frequent nocturnal voiding with or without excessive nocturnal urine production. The International Continence Society (ICS) has defined nocturia as waking up to pass urine twice or more each night. This classification of nocturia is referring to the number of micturitions as two or more nocturnal voids, regardless of the amount of urine produced during night time. Another proposed definition of nocturia might be "the event of a sleep disturbing voiding" (SDV).

The nocturnal micturition pattern varies with age. Newborn and infants void only during wakefulness or during arousal from sleep. Micturition never occurs during quiet sleep (Yeung 1995). In childhood sleep disturbing voiding disappears and is most often present as nocturnal enuresis. During teenage sleep disturbing voiding returns. Among children aged 7–12 fluid load shortly before bedtime in the younger age groups caused enuresis episodes as well as nocturia (Kirk et al. 1996), but after a certain age the response to bladder filling at night consistently was waking up and nocturia. Water-loading young people older than 15 years of age solely provoke nocturia (Hunsballe et al. 1995). During old age sleep disturbing voiding becomes extremely frequent.

3.   Prevalence of nocturia

Nocturia is almost equally frequent in men and women, but studies of nocturia are performed predominantly in men. There are not many reports about the mechanisms behind nocturia in women, so for the time being the hypothesis is the same for men and women. Overall prevalence of nocturia in men over 45 years of age is 56.1% ranging from 29.9% at the age of 45 to 81.8% at 90 years or older (Malmsten et al. 1997). In another study the prevalence rose from 66% to 91% in men aged 50–59 and 80+ years respectively (Middelkoop et al. 1996) and yet another study revealed a rise in the prevalence of nocturia from 16% in those aged 40–49 to 55% in those aged over 70 (Chute et al. 1993). The prevalence of female nocturia varies in the different reports from 3.3% to 93%. The 3.3% were elderly women of 75 years or more having to void three or more times during the night (Glenning 1985), whereas the 93% were elderly incontinent women with nocturnal voids of 1 or more (Barker and Mitteness 1988). In the International Continence Society – study of lower urinary tract symptoms in men 74% of the patients aged 60–69 years reported an average of two or more nocturnal voids (Peters et al. 1997).

4.   Impact of nocturia

The impact of nocturia on morbidity and mortality depends of the severity of the problem. It is a very distressing symptom and disrupted sleep reduces sleep quality, with impaired productivity and day-time fatigue. Studies of the impact of sleep quality have shown significant effects on both morbidity and mortality (Morgan et al. 1979, von Diest 1990, Windgard and Berkman 1983). Particularly in elderly people the risk of night time accidents increases, which may reduce life quality (Stewart et al. 1992).

5.   Aetiology

Variation in urine production during 24 hours is highly complex. Many factors are involved besides sleep habits and age. These include intravascular volume and pressure, renal perfusion, serum osmolality, and the level and activity of circulating hormones such as renin, angiotensin II, aldosterone, catecholamines, atrial natriuretic peptide (ANP), and argenine vasopressin (AVP) (Donahue and Lowenthal 1997).

It is important to distinguish between nocturnal polyuria (>35% of daily urine volume), which occurs despite a total daily urine volume that does not increase (Kirkland et al. 1983, Larsson and Victor 1988) and nocturnal frequency.

5.1   Nocturnal polyuria

Inappropriate fluid intake and use of agents with diuretic-like actions (alcohol) can in some cases explain a high nocturnal urine production. Besides these behavioural factors many medical conditions may disturb normal circadian urine output (Fig. 1) (Donahue and Lowenthal 1997). Also the use of diuretics may explain nocturnal polyuria. In these conditions the increased nocturnal diuresis is independent of vasopressin levels.

The antidiuretic hormone is one of the more important hormones responsible for the circadian variations in urine production. In childhood, production of AVP is very stable during daytime. During nighttime the hormone release peaks and lowers urine production. In teenagers the rhythm is not as pronounced as it was during childhood, and in adults the profile is even flatter, and in old age the profile is completely flat, leading to nighttime polyuria.

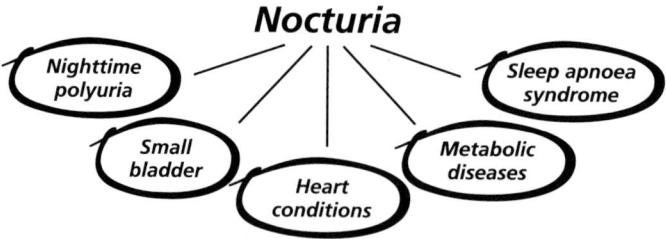

Fig. 1. Aetiology. Conditions disturbing normal circadian urine output

The group of patients with nocturnal polyuria is the enuretic children. These children have an average level of AVP in the daytime similar to normal levels. However, AVP levels fail to double at night in enuretic children as it does in children without enuresis (Rittig et al. 1989). The nocturnal polyuria syndrome (NPS) is characterised by an increased urine output during the night and consequently an increase in the nocturnal voiding frequency (Asplund 1995). It is thought to be caused by insufficient release of the antidiuretic hormone (AVP) during the night in otherwise healthy people.

Some studies among elderly persons show that plasma AVP concentration is higher in men than in women (Olsson et al. 1989). In one of these studies women had AVP levels that were only half or one third of those in men. They had no nocturnal increase in AVP irrespective of nocturnal voiding, whereas the men without nocturnal micturition showed a substantial increase in plasma AVP (Asplund and Aberg 1991).

A study of the pattern of urine flow and electrolyte excretion in healthy elderly people showed a reduction in day to night ratios of urinary excretion in older patients. They excrete more sodium, potassium, creatinine, and water over night than during daytime (Kirkland et al. 1983).

In a study of elderly men complaining of nocturia, some with nocturnal polyuria, and others with a normal nocturnal urine production a disturbed circadian rhythm of AVP was found. These men had no raise in AVP levels during evening and nighttime independent of nocturnal urine production. The group of men was compared with a healthy control group. The subgroup of patients with normal nocturnal urine production turned out to have the same profile in urine production, arterial blood pressure (ABP), and excretion of sodium as the control group. Only the functional bladder capacity (FBC) was significantly smaller than in the control group (Fig. 2). On the contrary the subgroup of patients with nocturnal polyuria had a tendency to have a

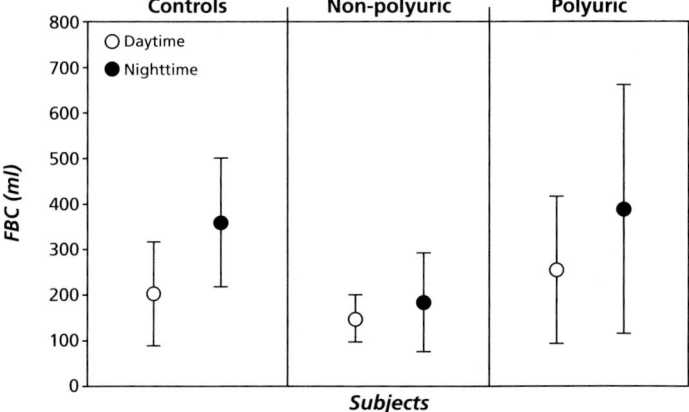

Fig. 2. The night- and daytime bladder capacity in elderly men with LUTS and a matched control group adapted from the PhD thesis "Pathophysiological aspects of nocturia" (T. B. Matthiesen, Aarhus University 1998)

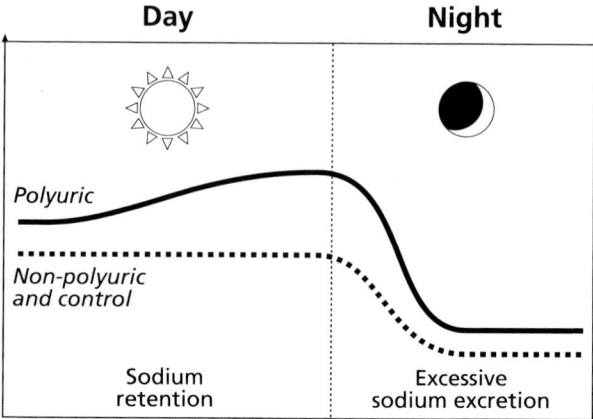

Fig. 3. Schematic drawing of the mean arterial blood pressure during 24-hours in elderly men with LUTS and controls. The solid line representing the polyurics and the dashed line representing non-polyurics and controls. During daytime the polyurics retained sodium leading to excessive sodium excretion during nighttime. This figure was modified from Matthiesen et al. J Urol 1996; 156: 1296 (Fig. 4)

slightly higher ABP in the afternoon and to accumulate sodium, leading to a sodium excreting polyuria during nighttime (Fig. 3) (Matthiesen et al. 1996). No significant differences were found between the groups in any of the measured hormones (AVP, ANP, angiotensin II, aldosterone).

Obviously the sensitivity to the antidiuretic hormone changes with age, and fluid regulation is taken over to some extent by other mechanisms.

5.2 Lower urinary tract symptoms (LUTS) and nocturnal frequency

It is well known that both men and women with age experience troublesome symptoms from the lower urinary tract. These can be due to detrusor overactivity, bladder hypersensitivity, or neurological disease with a small functional bladder capacity. Among elderly men an enlarged prostate can cause incomplete bladder emptying and irritative symptoms that often results in nocturnal frequency.

Especially around menopause many women experience LUTS. In addition to the above-mentioned conditions the women also report symptoms of stress incontinence, nocturia, and irritative symptoms such as dysuria, urgency, frequency, and urinary tract infections (Cardozo and Kelleher 1995). Already existing symptoms often become worse when the women enter the menopause.

5.3 Sleep disorders

Sleep disorders are common in elderly people, and often the cause of waking up from sleep. The high incidence of both nocturia and sleep disorders such as sleep apnoea in elderly people and other patients suggests that sleep disorders may be the cause of some awakenings from sleep rather than nocturia. In a sleep study only 5% of the patients correctly identified the source of their awakening from sleep. Most of awakenings from sleep attributed by the patients to be pressure to urinate were instead a result of sleep disorder (Pressman et al. 1996). Sleep apnoea leads to a high intra-thoracic pressure which stimulates atrial natriuretic peptide (ANP) production and by that a high nocturnal urine production.

6. Treatment

A thorough investigation of the patient is crucial to be able to initiate effective treatment of any urological symptom including nocturia. Diaries and pad weighing tests are important tools to decide whether nocturia is caused by nocturnal polyuria and/or a small bladder. Naturally the treatment is dependent on the aetiology of the condition. In many medical conditions well documented and effective treatments are already available.

6.1 Reduction of nocturnal urine production

In the group of otherwise healthy people with nocturnal polyuria and consequently nocturnal frequency the treatment must be targeted towards lowering the nocturnal urine production. Diuretics in the afternoon will in some cases dry up the patient and thereby reduce the nocturnal diuresis. Furosemide taken 6 hours before bedtime reduces night time frequency and voided volume significantly (Reynard et al. 1998).

Alterations of drinking habits towards restricted fluid intake during the evening will of cause decrease nocturnal diuresis and nocturnal frequency.

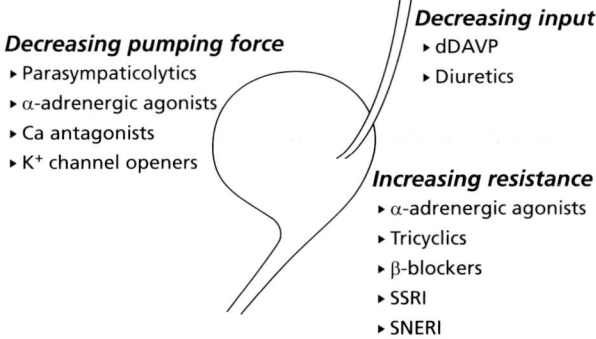

Decreasing pumping force
▸ Parasympaticolytics
▸ α-adrenergic agonists
▸ Ca antagonists
▸ K⁺ channel openers

Decreasing input
▸ dDAVP
▸ Diuretics

Increasing resistance
▸ α-adrenergic agonists
▸ Tricyclics
▸ β-blockers
▸ SSRI
▸ SNERI

Fig. 4. Treatment modalities of the primary urological condition leading to nocturia either via decreasing urinary output, decreasing the pumping force (modelling the detrusor activity) or increasing urethral resistance

Also the type of fluid intake seems to be important. A vasopressin insensitive state may be caused by ethanol (Denker and Brenner 1998) resulting in a polyuric state. Caffeine-rich fluids such as coffee and cola increase smooth muscle contractility (Lee et al. 1993), which may aggravate already existing detrusor instability (Arya et al. 2000) so the patient experiences a worsening of frequency.

The synthetic vasopressin analogue desmopressin acetate is an anti-diuretic agent and effective in lowering urine production (Asplund and Aberg 1993, Hilton and Stanton 1982). The duration of action of the drug is usually fairly long and, as with AVP, the sensitivity to desmo-pressin seems to be increasing with age. Therefore precaution must be taken when desmopressin is given to elderly persons (Carter et al. 1992) (Fig. 4).

6.2   Frequency without nocturnal polyuria

An agent that helps the detrusor muscle to relax and enables the bladder to contain more urine before emptying is the treatment of choice in the group of people complaining of nocturnal frequency without any signs of nocturnal polyuria.

Antispasmolytic agents may be able to restrain such uncontrolled bladder contractions but also reducing the nocturnal urine output seems to help this group (Hilton and Stanton 1982). Anticholinergic drugs increase the volume at which the first unstable detrusor contraction is triggered, decrease the strength of the contraction, and thereby increase the bladder capacity. Unfortunately the anticholinergic side effects are often proble-matic and may limit patient compliance.

Also oestrogen replacement seems to alleviate the symptoms of urgency, urge incontinence, frequency, and nocturia in women (Cardozo and Kelleher 1995). Combined therapy is often necessary to achieve acceptable results (Fig. 4).

7.   Closing remarks

With increased focus on quality of life and an almost explosive increase in the number of elderly persons especially in Western societies, it is no wonder that nocturia has been brought into focus. Nocturia does not only disturb sleep, it can be associated with serious pathologies, or it may by itself lead to pathology.

So far, there are still a number of questions remaining regarding nocturia, and the treatment options are fewer than desirable. We have highlighted some of the aspects of nocturia and have suggested a more global nomen-clature by the introduction of the term sleep disturbing voiding. We will no doubt over the next decades experience an intensified focus on both the pathogenesis and the treatment of the condition.

List of abbreviations

LUTS	Lower Urinary Tract Symptoms
BOO	Bladder Outlet Obstruction
ICS	International Continence Society
SDV	Sleep Disturbing Voiding
ANP	Atrial Natriuretic Peptide
AVP	Argenine Vasopressin
NPS	Nocturnal Polyuria Syndrome
ABP	Arterial Blood Pressure
FBC	Functional Bladder Capacity

8.   References

1. Asplund R (1995) The nocturnal polyuria syndrome (NPS). Gen Pharmacol 26(6): 1203–1209
2. Asplund R, Aberg H (1991) Diurnal variation in the levels of anti-diuretic hormone in the elderly. J Intern Med 229(2): 131–134
3. Asplund R, Aberg HE (1992) Micturition habits of older people. Scand J Urol Nephrol 26: 345–349
4. Asplund R, Aberg H (1993) Desmopressin in elderly subjects with increased nocturnal diuresis. A two-month treatment study. Scand J Urol Nephrol 27(1): 77–82
5. Ayra LA, Myers DL, Jackson ND (2000) Dietary caffeine intake and the risk for detrusor instability: a case-control study. Obstet Gynecol 96(1): 85–89
6. Barker JC, Mitteness LS (1988) Nocturia in the elderly. Gerontologist 28(1): 99–104
7. Cardozo LD, Kelleher CJ (1995) Sex hormones, the menopause and urinary problems. Gynecol Endocrinol 9(1): 75–84
8. Carter PG, Cannon AA, McConnell, Abrams P (1999) Role of atrial natriuretic peptide in nocturnal polyuria in elderly males. European Urology 36(3): 213–220
9. Carter PG, McConnell AA, Abrams P (1992) The safety and efficacy of dDAVP in the elderly. Neurourol Urol 11: 421–422
10. Chute CG, Panser LA, Girman CJ, Oesterling JE, Guess HA, Jacobsen SJ, Lieber MM (1993) The prevalence of prostatism: A population-based survey of urinary symptoms. J Urol 150(1): 85–89
11. Denker BM, Brenner BM (1998) Alterations in urinary function and electrolytes. In: Fauci AS, Braunwald E, Isselbacher KJ (eds) Harrison's principles of internal medicine. MacGraw-Hill: New York, pp 261–262
12. Diokno AC, Brown MB, Brock BM, Herzog AR, Normolle DP (1988) Clinical and cystometric characteristics of continent and incontinent noninstitutionalized elderly. J Urol 140: 567–571
13. Donahue JL, Lowenthal DT (1997) Nocturnal polyuria in the elderly person. AM J Med Sci 314(4): 232–238
14. Glenning PP (1985) Urinary voiding patterns of apparently normal Women. Aust NZ J Obstet Gynaec 25(1): 62–65
15. Hald T, Horn T (1998) The human urinary bladder in aging. Br J Urol 82 [Suppl 1]: 59–64
16. Hilton P, Stanton SL (1982) The use of desmopressin (DDAVP) in nocturnal urinary frequency in the female. Br J Urol 54(3): 252–255

17. Hunsballe JM, Hansen TK, Rittig S, Norgaard JP, Pedersen EB, Djurhuus JC (1995) Polyuric and non-polyuric bedwetting-pathogenic differences in nocturnal enuresis. Scand J Urol Nephrol [Suppl] 173: 77–78

18. Kirk J, Rasmussen PV, Rittig S, Djurhuus JC (1996) Provoked enuresis-like episodes in healthy children 7 to 12 years old. J Urol 156(1): 210–213

19. Kirkland JL, Lye M, Levy DW, Banerjee AK (1983) Pattern of urine flow and electrolyte excretion in healthy elderly people. BMJ 287: 1665–1667

20. Larsson G, Victor A (1988) Micturition patterns in a healthy female population, studied with a frequency/volume chart. Scand J Urol Nephrol [Suppl] 114: 53–57

21. Lee JG, Wein AJ, Levin RM (1993) The effects of caffeine on the contractile response of the rabbit urinary bladder to field stimulation. Gen Pharmacol 24(4): 1007–1011

22. Malmsten UG, Milsom I, Molander U, Norlen LJ (1997) Urinary incontinence and lower urinary tract symptoms: An epidemiological study of men aged 45 to 99 years. J Urol 158(5): 1733–1737

23. Matthiesen TB, Rittig S, Norgaard JP, Pedersen EB, Djurhuus JC (1996) Nocturnal polyuria and natriuresis in male patients with nocturia and lower urinary tract symptoms. J Urol 156(4): 1292–1299

24. Middelkoop HA, Smilde-van dDD, Neven AK, Kamphuisen HA, Springer CP (1996) Subjective sleep characteristics of 1,485 males and females aged 50–93: Effects of sex and age, and factors related to self-evaluated quality of sleep. J Gerontol 51(3): M108–M115

25. Morgan K, Healey DW, Healey PJ (1989) Factors influencing persistent subjective insomnia in old age: a follow up study of good and poor sleepers aged 65–74. Age Aging 18(2): 117–122

26. Olsson T, Viitanen M, Hagg E, Asplund K, Grankvist K, Eriksson S, Gustafson Y (1989) Hormones in 'young' and 'old' elderly: Pituitary-thyroid and pituitary-adrenal axes. Gerontology 35(2–3): 144–152

27. Peters TJ, Donovan JL, Kay HE, Abrams P, de la Rosette JJMCH, Porru D, Thuroff JW (1997) The International Continence Society "benign prostatic hyperplasia", study: The bothersomeness of urinary symptoms. J Urol 157: 885–889

28. Pressman MR, Figueroa WG, Kendrick-Mohamed J, Greenspon LW, Peterson DD (1996) Nocturia. A rarely recognized symptom of sleep apnea and other occult sleep disorders. Arch Intern Med 156(5): 545–550

29. Rembratt A, Robertson GL, Norgaard JP, Andersson KE (2000) Pathogenic aspects of nocturia in the elderly: Differences between nocturics and non-nocturics. ICS meeting

30. Resnick NM (1988) Voiding dysfunction in the elderly. In: Yalla SV, McGuire EJ, Elbadawi A, Blaivas JG (eds) Neurourology and urodynamics. Principle and practice. Macmillan: New York, pp 303–330

31. Resnick NM (1990) Noninvasive diagnosis of the patient with complex incontinence. Gerontology [Suppl] 2: 8–18

32. Resnick NM, Elbadawi A, Yalla SV (1995) Age and the lower urinary tract: what is normal? Neurourol Urodyn 14: 577–579

33. Reynard JM, Cannon A, Yang Q, Abrams P (1998) A double-blind randomized trial of frusemide against placebo. Br J Urol 81(2): 215–218

34. Rittig S, Knudsen UB, Jolner M, Norgaard JP, Pedersen EB, Djurhuus JC (1989) Adult enuresis. The role of vasopressin and atrial natriuretic peptide. Scand J Urol Nephrol [Suppl] 125: 79–86

35. Rittig S, Knudsen UB, Norgaard JP, Pedersen EB, Djurhuus JC (1989) Abnormal diurnal rhythm of plasma vasopressin and urinary output in patients with enuresis. Am J Physiol 256(4 Pt 2): F664–F671

36. Robertson GL, Rittig S, Kovacs L, Gaskill MB, Zee P, Naninga J (1999) Pathophysiology and treatment of enuresis in adults. Scand J Urol Nephrol [Suppl] 202: 36–39

37. Rodger RSC (1998) Renal function in the elderly. Br J Urol 82 [Suppl 1]: 65–70

38. Stewart RB, Moore MT, May FE, Marks RG, Hale WE (1992) Nocturia: A risk factor for falls in the elderly. J Am Geriatr Soc 40(12): 1217–1220

39. von Diest R (1990) Subjective sleep characteristics as coronary risk factor, their association with type A behavior and vital exhaustion. J Psychosom Res 34: 415

40. Windgard DL, Berkman PT (1983) Mortality risk associated with sleeping patterns among adults. Sleep 6: 102

41. Yeung CK (1995) The normal infant bladder. Scand J Urol Nephrol [Suppl] 173: 19–23

Correspondence address: J. C. Djurhuus, MD, DMSc, International Enuresis Research Center, Institute of Experimental Clinical Research, Skejby Hospital, DK-8200 Aarhus, Denmark (E-mail: jcd@iekf.au.dk).

Impact of central nervous system alterations to bladder dysfunction in elderly people

M. Schmidbauer

Department of Neurology, Lainz Hospital, Vienna, Austria

Contents

1.   Introduction

Regardless of 150 years of progression in the neurosciences, neurogenic control of micturation is not fully understood. This is due to the methods of research in correlative neurology, which are not in all instances satisfactory for defining central vegetative control functions, including the mechanisms involved in bladder control:

- A "nucleus" composed of grey matter has to be localized exactly whenever stimulation is intended to uncover its function or ablation is intended to erase function. This is possible only when a nucleus is well delineated but not possible in diffusely circumscribed grey masses.
- Fibre degeneration following a lesion is an approach to the interconnections between respective nuclei or other circumscribed areas of grey matter. By using this "Wallerian" degeneration, efferent fibre tracts can be traced from a damaged area of origin to the target area as far as a representative proportion

of fibres are well myelinated, since myelin breakdown products subserve as "tracers" along the course of degenerating fibres. Clinical case studies are commonly based on this "lesion method" and Wallerian degeneration.
- Experimental tracer studies and transmitter mapping are further main tools in the general spectrum of neuroscientific research.

With regard to the central nervous control of bladder function, many problems remain beyond the scope of this approach:

- Many components in the network of bladder control are located in the brainstem and form part of the reticular formation (RF) (Nieuwenhuys et al. 1988). They are loosely scattered arrangements of nerve cells, by no means sharply demarcated, definite nuclei, and they exhibit multidirected fibre connections as the common hallmark of systems subserving multimodal integration. Their fibres are typically thin and mainly unmyelinated (Nieuwenhuys et al. 1998). They are therefore not suitable for the lesion method using Wallerian degeneration.
- Stimulation with microelectrodes or ablation in animal models are rather unselective when the anatomical target to electrode insertion is indistinct.
- Clinical tests on bladder function in acute CNS lesions are hampered, when permanent catheters in patients are necessary due to impaired consciousness or the need of permanent fluid balance control.
- Pharmacological side effects of various individual medications on bladder function is a routine problem (Müller-Oerlinghausen et al. 1999).
- Studies on human lesions are often restricted to rare cases; impacts on general conclusions are doubtful.

Table 1. Central nervous system structures affiliated to bladder function (according to Appenzeller)

	Support of bladder contraction	Support of bladder relaxation
Telencephalon	Caudal Gyrus cinguli Caudal Cingulum	
Diencephalon	Lateral/caudal Hypothalamus Stria terminalis Commissura anterior Nucleus Praeopticus Ventral septum	Caudal Hypothalamus
Mesencephalon	Colliculus superior Area intercollicularis Central gray matter Tegmental RF	Vicinity of contraction supporting mesencephalic area
Pons	Dorsolateral RF	Ventrolateral RF
Medulla oblongata	Bulbar center of bladder contraction, tegmentum	Bulbar center of bladder relaxation, tegmentum
Cerebellum	Nucleus fastigii Nucleus globosus Nucleus emboliformis	

- Agents with selective action on "transmitter systems" are not simply probes of *one* function since any neuromodulator may act in an excitatory or inhibitory manner, depending on the area that is taken into account. (Nieuwenhuys et al. 1998).
- Correlative studies in anatomy and physiology show that in the diencephalon, the mesencephalon, the pons, and the medulla oblongata, areas with bladder contracting impact are co-localised with bladder relaxing areas (see Tables 1–4, according to Appenzeller 1990). Thus, clinical lesions in humans often affect both agonistic and antagonistic areas, with varying proportions in the resulting impairment of function.

Table 2. Descending pathways supporting bladder contraction from supraspinal areas

TRACT (tr.)	Tr. tectobulbaris & fasciculus long. dorsalis	Along with tr. rubrospinalis – tr. reticulospinalis lateralis	Tr. reticulospinalis ventralis & lateralis
Origin	Mesencephalon	Mesencephalon Pontine detrusor – nucleus Bulbar contraction center	Bulbar contraction center
Target	Bulbar relaxation – contraction center	Lumbosacral lateral columns Sacral anterior horns	Sacral micturation center

Table 3. Descending pathways supporting bladder relaxation from supraspinal areas

Tract	Along with fasciculus long. medialis – tractus reticulospinalis medialis	Tr. reticulospinalis ventralis
Origin	Pontine relaxation center	Bulbar relaxation center
Target	Sacral spinal anterior horn	Sacral micturition center
Function	Contraction of the external urethral sphincter	Inhibition of detrusor, bladder relaxation

Table 4. Ascending pathways from the sacral micturation centers

Tract	"Pelvine sensory vagus"	Tr. sacrobulbaris
Origin	Nervus pudendus Nervi pelvini	Lateral columns of sacral – and coccygeal segments
Target	Medulla oblongata, thalamus	Rostral Nucleus gracilis
Function	Propagation of stretching impulses from the bladder?	"Pelvico – abdominal reflex"

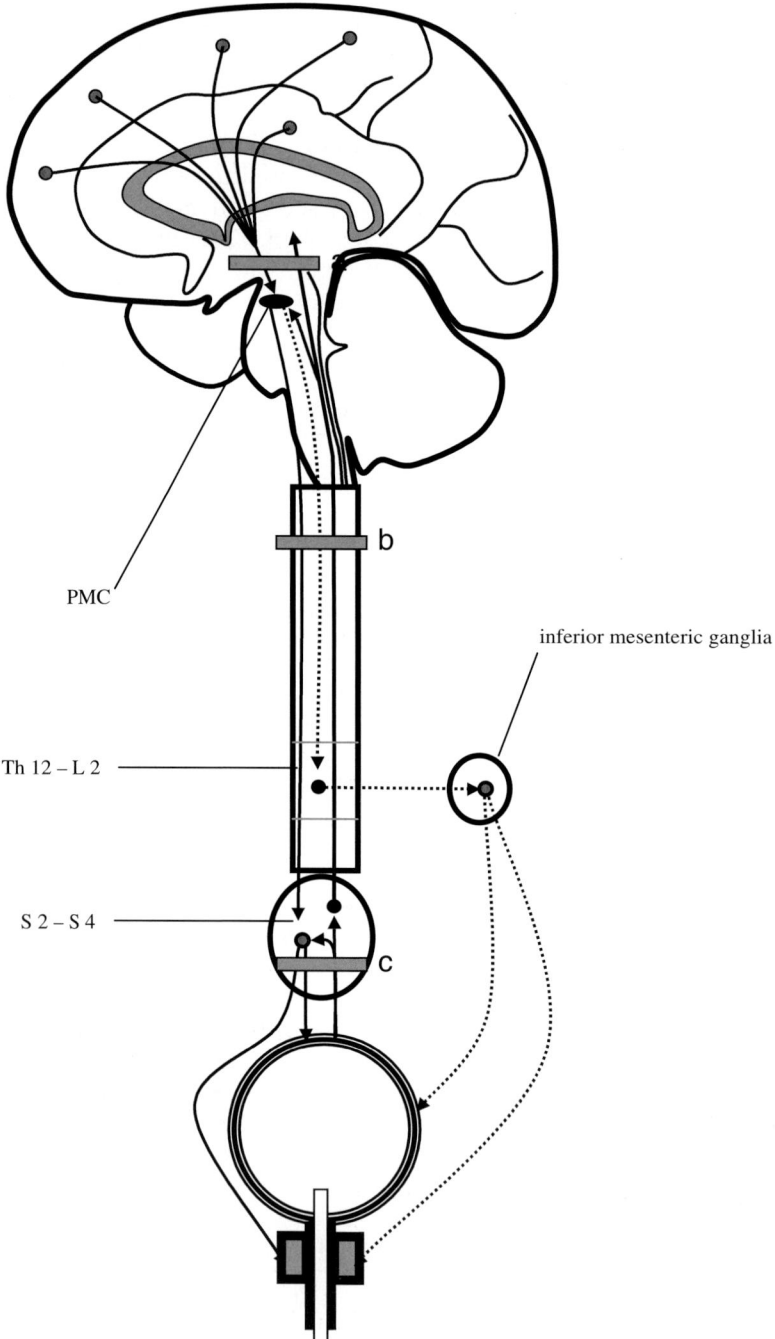

PMC

inferior mesenteric ganglia

Th 12 – L 2

S 2 – S 4

Fig. 1. Schematic diagram of some clinically relevant CNS structures thought to be involved in the control of micturation (represented with permission from Paur and Schmidbauer)

However, three main patterns of CNS related bladder dysfunction can be outlined: a. detrusor overactivity/urge incontinence, b. reflex dyssynergia, and c. areflexia/hyporeflexia of the detrusor, corresponding to suprapontine lesions (a), lesions between the pontine and sacral centres of micturation in the spinal cord (b), and lesions of the sacral centres for micturation or the peripheral nerves (c) (Fig. 1).

The anatomical sites as detailed in Tables 1–4 do not strictly represent respective areas of bladder control. They serve as approximate topographical landmarks and give a preliminary summary of heterogeneous results from various neuroscientific methods.

2. Patterns of bladder dysfunction due to diseases of the central nervous system

2.1 Detrusor overactivity/urge incontinence

Symptoms associated with lesions above the "pontine micturition centre"

Urgency	+
Frequent urination	+
Retention	−
Stress incontinence	+
Reflex contractions	+
Overflow incontinence	−
Urinary flow	**normal**

2.2 Reflex dyssynergia

Symptoms associated with lesions between the pontine and the sacral micturition centres

Urgency	+
Frequent urination	+
Retention	+
Stress incontinence	+
Reflex contractions	+
Overflow incontinence	−
Urinary flow	**reduced**

2.3 Detrusor hyporeflexia/areflexia

Symptoms associated with lesions of the sacral micturition centre or peripheral nerves

Urgency	–
Frequent urination	+/–
Retention	+
Stress incontinence	+
Reflex contractions	–
Overflow incontinence	+
Urinary flow	**reduced**

3. Diseases of the central nervous system associated with voiding dysfunction

3.1 Detrusor overactivity/urge incontinence

3.1.1 *Subcortical vascular encephalopathy/"Small vessel disease"*

The indicative neuropathology consists of fibrohyalinosis and segmental dissociation of arterioles and small to medium sized arteries (Fig. 2a) in the white matter of the brain, the basal ganglia, the thalamus, and, less constantly, the pons, due to arterial hypertension and diabetes mellitus.

Functional results are an impairment of microcirculation and extravasation of plasma, leading to circumscribed elective or total micronecroses of tissue. The typical correlative finding in computed tomography and magnetic resonance imaging of the brain is a diffuse white matter damage, so called leucoaraiosis (Fig. 2b) and lacunar infarctions, particularly in the basal ganglia and in the thalamus (Ginsberg and Bogousslavsky 1998).

Dependent on the respective functional significance of the area of damage, either a diffuse progressive or a recurrent apoplectiform clinical course may occur. This leads to a progressive decline in motor, cognitive, and memory functions, combined with transient focal signs (Ginsberg and Bogousslavsky 1998).

Since the main impact of pathology is focused above the pons, the typical bladder dysfunction in this condition is a detrusor overactivity/urge incontinence.

3.1.2 *Parkinson's disease*

The indicative neuropathology with Lewy bodies (Fig. 3a), nerve cell loss, and gliosis does not only affect the substantia nigra but may also diffusely involve the cerebral cortex, the diencephalon, the lateral columns of the spinal cord, sympathetic and parasympathetic ganglia (Markesbery 1998). The clinical pattern consists of initially asymmetric akinetic or rigid dysfunction of the limbs, hypomimic face expression, and tremor at rest. These classical signs are combined with, or followed by, cognitive decline and vegetative impairments (Calne 1994).

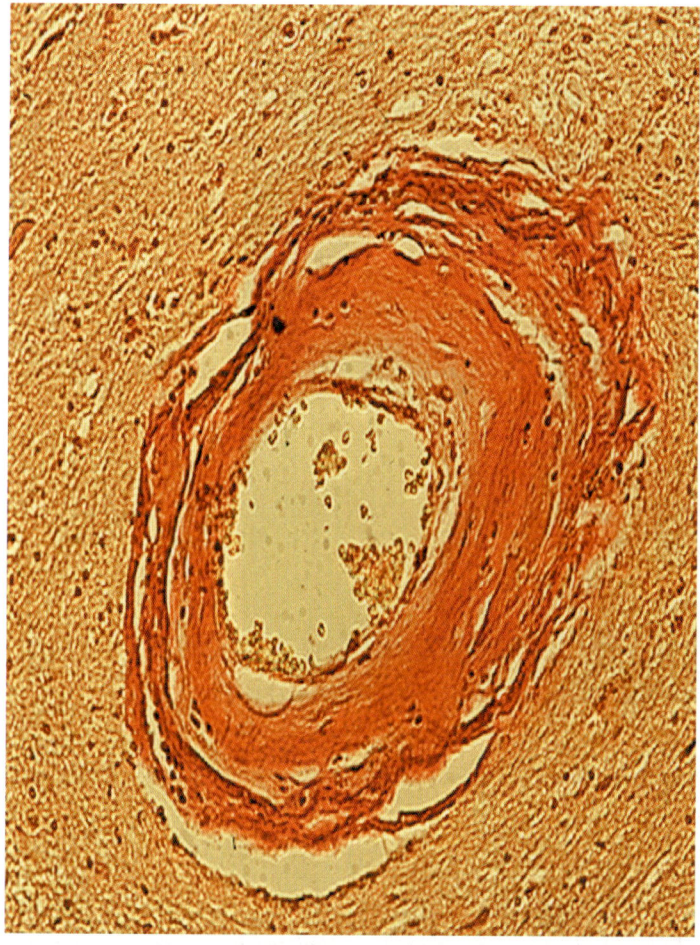

a

Fig. 2a. Segmental dissociation in a small fibrohyalinotic blood vessel, due to arterial hypertension (Gieson Elastica × 20)

According to the wide extension of the pathology, bladder dysfunction differs in individual presentation. The main patterns are the detrusor overactivity/urge incontinence and the areflexia/hyporeflexia of the detrusor.

3.1.3 Alzheimer's disease

A characteristic sequence in the occurrence of neurofibrillary tangles and senile plaques as histopathological hallmarks (Markesbery 1998) (Fig. 4a) is initiated in the allocortex of the temporal lobe and progresses to the parietal lobe and finally to the frontal lobe, causing atrophy (Fig. 4b). Other main sites of tissue destruction are the amygdala, the anterior parts of the thalamus, the cholinergic system of the basal forebrain, and parts of the

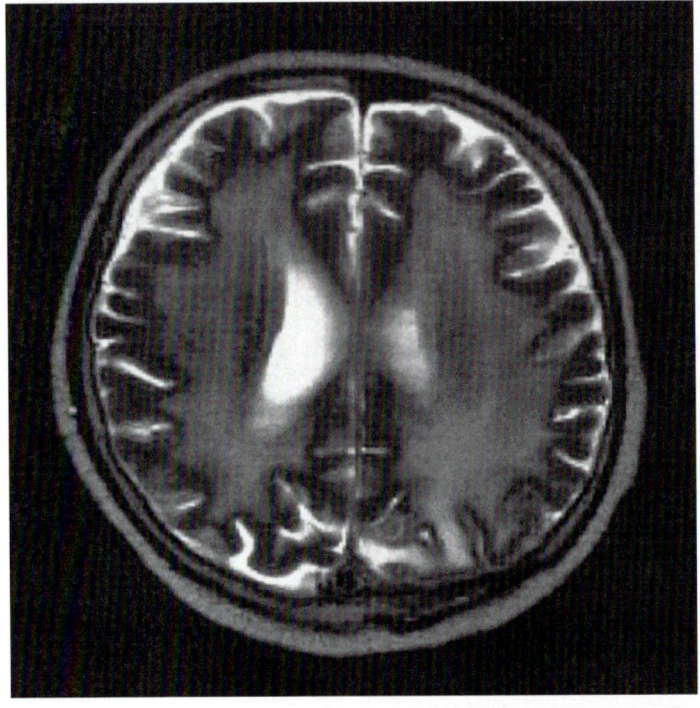

b

Fig. 2b. MRI-T2 weighted image of the brain with advanced leucoaraiosis in small vessel disease

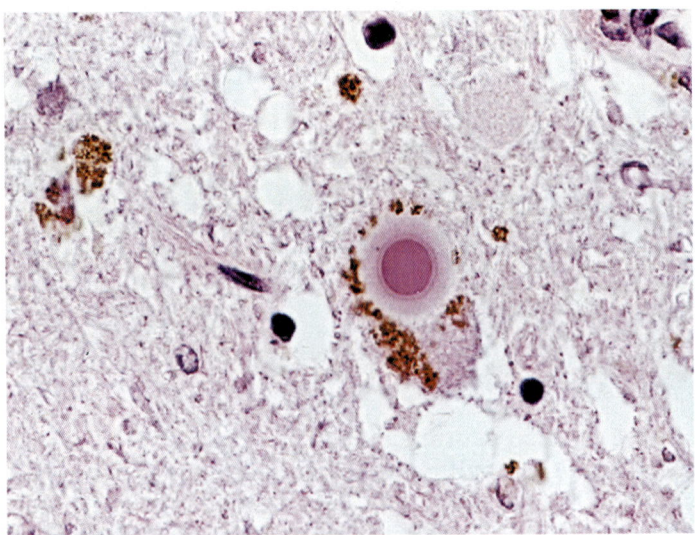

Fig. 3. Lewy – Body in the substantia nigra and spongiform tissue alteration (Hematoxylin Eosin × 100)

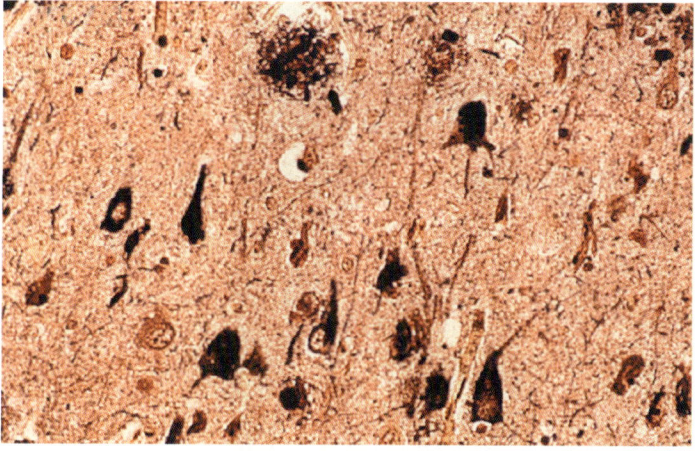

a

Fig. 4a. Neurofibrillary tangles and senile plaque in Alzheimer's disease (Bielschowsky silver stain × 40)

monoaminergic system such as the locus coeruleus and the raphe complex (Calne 1994). This correlates to a clinical sequence with initial impairment of episodic memory function, progressing to injury of space orientation capacity and further to a disintegration of the individual personality within few years. In advanced stages of the disease, functional tomography, i.e. positron emission tomography (PET) or single photon emission computed tomography (SPECT), exhibits a marked decline in metabolism of the temporal, parietal, and frontal lobes (Fig. 4c). The suprapontine concentration of neuropathology leads to a detrusor overactivity/urge incontinence.

3.1.4 Normal pressure hydrocephalus

The arterial pulse of the brain and the periodic changes of the venous pressure of the spinal system are the motors of circulation of cerebrospinal fluid (CSF) from the lateral ventricles to the base of the brain, with an ascending stream to the granulations of Pacchioni and a descending stream to the lumbar sac (Felgenhauer and Beuche 1999, Dawson et al. 1987). Extension of the ventricles (Fig. 5) due to an aqueduct stenosis or dynamic disturbances of CSF flow causes leakage of ependymal surface of the lateral ventricles and leads to CSF penetration into the subependymal white matter, resulting in oedema, fibre degeneration, and consecutive gliosis. A compensatory resorption of the CSF via the periventricular veins is the reason for stable pressure gradients in this condition.

The clinical presentation is a characteristic sequence of initial gait disturbance, cognitive decline and finally detrusor overactivity/urge incontinence.

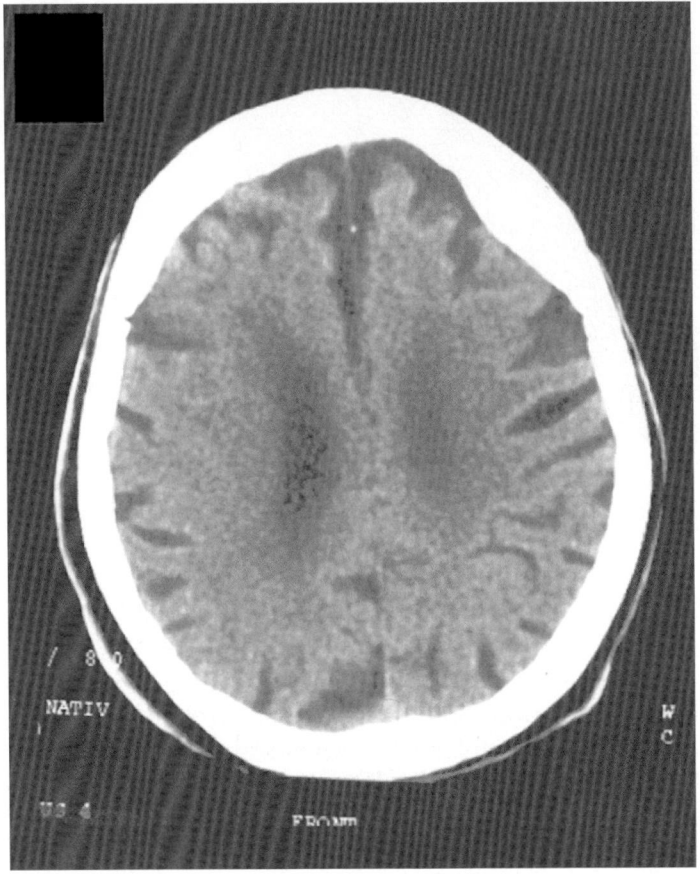

b

Fig. 4b. CT scan showing slight widening of the outer CSF space of the frontal lobe in Alzheimer's disease

3.2 Reflex dyssynergia

3.2.1 Cervical vertebrostenosis/chronic cord compression

In the spinal cord, impairment of the venous drainage and microcirculation is much more important than in the vascular pathology of the brain. This is because of tight safe longitudinal and transversal arterial anastomoses on the surface of the cord, which result in highly stable arterial blood supply, whereas the risk of compression is much higher due to the working motions of the spine/cord – complex and traction forces acting both on the spinal cord vessels and surrounding tissue.

Further, an increase of the intrathoracic or abdominal pressure may hamper venous drainage from the cord, and degenerative changes of the spine may cause stenosis of the spinal canal (Fig. 6). Thus, in elderly people, a broad spectrum of factors may cause compression of the spinal cord, such

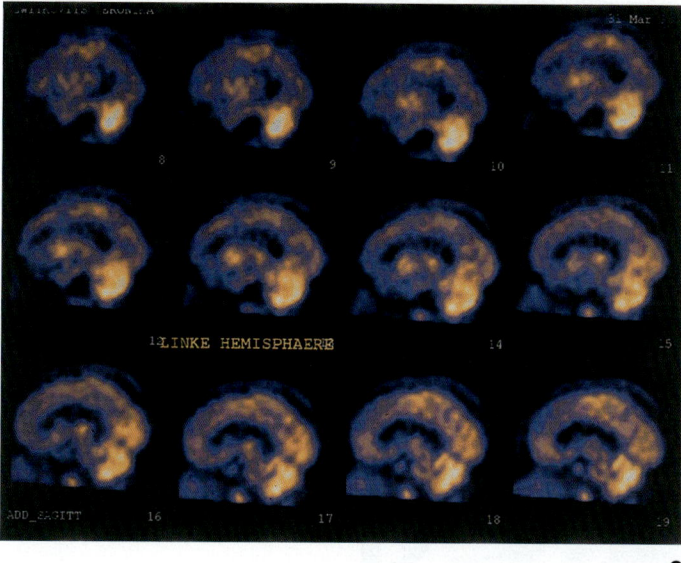

Fig. 4c. HMPAO – SPECT sagittal sections, indicating hypometabolism of the temporal, parietal and frontal lobes in Alzheimer's disease. Unimpaired tracer uptake is visible in the cerebellum

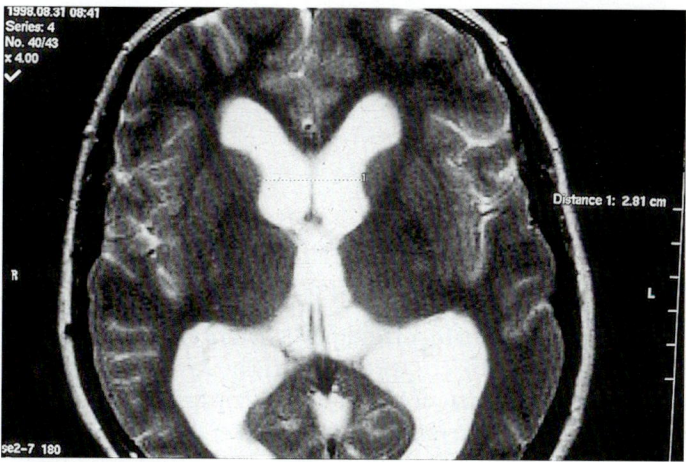

Fig. 5. MRI-T2 weighted image of the brain in normal pressure hydrocephalus with widening of the ventricles

as impairment of venous drainage, consecutive increases in tissue volume, increases in tissue pressure, and finally result in a breakdown of the local spinal microcirculation. Arterial factors play a minor part in this patho-genetic concert (Schneider 1980).

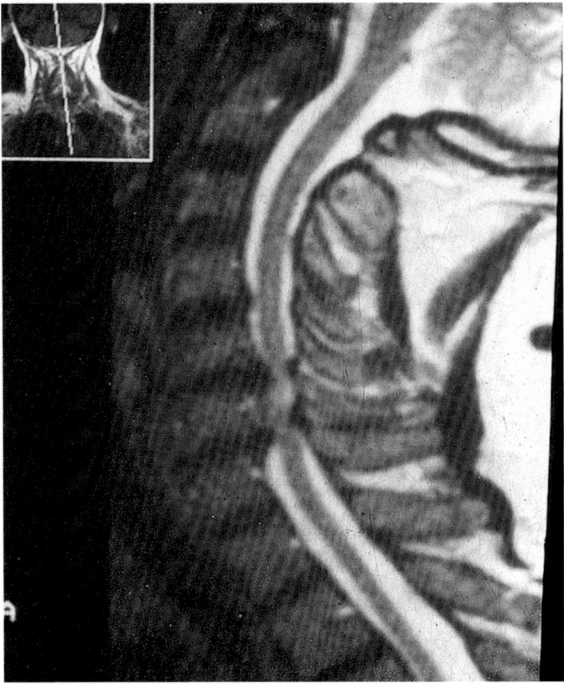

Fig. 6. MRI-T2 weighted image of the cervical spine with consumption of the spinal CSF space at the vertebral levels C5/6 and C6/7 due to stenosis of the spinal canal

Clinically it is presenting as chronic progressive motor impairment, leading to spastic paraparesis or tetraparesis, muscle atrophy, and minor sensory impairments. The concomitant bladder dysfunction results in reflex dyssynergia.

3.3 Hyporeflexia/areflexia of the detrusor

3.3.1 Lower spine vertebrostenosis/chronic cord compression

Lesions of the sacral micturition centre in elderly patients are frequently seen in Parkinson's disease (see above), compression to the lower spinal cord or cauda equina as an equivalent to cervical cord compression. These alterations can cause hyporeflexia or even areflexia of the detrusor.

4. Closing remarks

Changes in the filling and voiding phase of the bladder detrusor are common findings associated with diseases of the central nervous system. The combination of these central alterations with changes in detrusor function or an imbalance in detrusor-sphincter function can result in distressing symptoms for the patient. Therefore, an interdisciplinary diagnostic and therapeutic approach of urologists, neurologists and internal medicine specialists is recommended for the treatment of patients with neurological disease and voiding disorders. In addition to direct disease specific alterations of detrusor or sphincter innervation and function, several neurotropic medications frequently used in elderly people – such as antidepressants, neuroleptics, anticonvulsants, analgesic drugs and dopaminergic drugs, etc. – will improve neurologic symptoms but, concomitantly, aggravate voiding disorders.

5. References

1. Appenzeller O (1990) The autonomic nervous system – an introduction to basic and clinical concepts, 4th edn. Elsevier: Amsterdam, New York, Oxford
2. Calne DB (1994) Neurodegenerative diseases. W.B. Saunders Company: Philadelphia, London, Toronto, Montreal, Sydney, Tokyo
3. Dawson H, Welch K, Segal MB (1987) The physiology and pathophysiology of the cerebrospinal fluid. Churchill Livingstone: Edinburgh, London, Melbourne, New York
4. Felgenhauer K, Beuche W (1999) Labordiagnostik neurologischer Erkrankungen (Liquoranalytik und – zytologie, Diagnose – und Prozessmarker). Georg Thieme: Stuttgart, New York
5. Ginsberg MD, Bogousslavsky J (1998) Cerebrovascular disease. Pathophysiology, diagnosis, and management. Blackwell Science: USA
6. Markesbery WR (1998) Neuropathology of dementing disorders. Hodder Arnold: London, New York, Sydney, Auckland
7. Müller-Oerlinghausen B, Lasek R, Düppenbecker H, Munter KH (1999) Handbuch der unerwünschten Arzneimittelwirkungen. Urban & Fischer: München, Jena
8. Nieuwenhuys R, Ten Donkelaar HJ, Nicholson C (1998) The central nervous system of vertebrates. Springer: Berlin, Heidelberg, New York, Tokyo
9. Nieuwenhuys R, Voogd J, van Huijzen C (1988) The human central nervous system – a synopsis and atlas, 3rd edn. Springer: Berlin, Heidelberg
10. Schneider H (1980) Kreislaufstörungen und Gefäßprozesse des Rückenmarks. In: Ule G, Doerr W, Seifert G, Uehlinger E (eds) Pathologie des Nervensystems; Band 13/1 Spezielle Pathologische Anatomie. Springer: Berlin, Heidelberg, New York

Correspondence address: Manfred Schmidbauer, MD, Department of Neurology, Lainz Hospital, Wolkersbergenstrasse 1, A-1130 Vienna, Austria (E-mail: manfred.schmidbauer@wienkav.at).

Urodynamic findings in aging people

F. Trigo Rocha, C. Mendes Gomes, and *S. Arap*

Division of Urology, University of São Paulo School of Medicine,
São Paulo, Brazil

Contents

1.   Introduction

Lower urinary tract dysfunction is a major cause of morbidity and decreased quality of life in elderly men and women. A number of studies have shown that the prevalence and bothersomeness of lower urinary tract symptoms (LUTS) increase with age (Hampel et al. 1997, Haidinger et al. 1999, Koskimaki et al. 1998). Urinary incontinence is the most common problem and is reported to affect 15–35% of community dwelling individuals and 22–90% of residents in nursing homes (Fantl et al. 1996, Schmidbauer et al. 2001, Chiarelli and Brown 1999, Damian et al. 1998). Despite these figures, many patients avoid discussing their problems with family members or health care professionals for being too embarrassed or having low expectations of treatment (Rovner et al. 2002, Roberts et al. 1998). Many doctors do not investigate their patients' urinary problems. This situation is unfortunate as with proper evaluation much can be done to alleviate lower urinary tract symptoms. Moreover, complications may arise from neglected or improperly treated voiding dysfunction, including urinary tract infections, urinary retention, and even upper urinary tract damage.

The evaluation of elderly people with LUTS requires a thorough understanding of the voiding physiology as well as the pathophysiological changes associated with aging. Most urinary problems in the elderly are multifactorial in origin, demanding a comprehensive assessment of the organs of the lower urinary tract, functional impairments, and concurrent medical diseases. Even in the absence of pathological conditions, the lower urinary tract changes as the individual ages. Detrusor contractility as well as bladder capacity and the ability to postpone voiding decline in both sexes, whereas urinary flow decreases with age. Benign prostatic hyperplasia (BPH) causes the prostate to enlarge in most men, causing infravesical obstruction in nearly 50% of them (Gomes et al. 2001, Resnick et al. 1995). Other important changes observed in elderly men and women are an increased prevalence of involuntary bladder contractions and increased post-void residual (PVR) volume (Hampel et al. 1997, Homma et al. 1994). Urinary output during night time is also increased even in the absence of congestive heart failure, BPH, or other medical conditions. This fact in association with the sleep disorders that are common in elderly people makes one or two episodes of nocturia a normal pattern in most healthy individuals in this age group. This chapter reviews the applications and findings of urodynamic studies in the elderly population. Detailed descriptions of the pathophysiology, clinical evaluation, and treatment of LUTS in elderly people are addressed in other chapters of this book. Technical aspects of the different urodynamic tests are also not addressed in this chapter and the interested reader will find numerous specialised books and periodics on that subject (Mundy et al. 1994, Nitti 1998, Boone 1996a, Boone 1996b).

2.   Clinical evaluation

Geriatric patients may present with a broad spectrum of mental and physical disabilities, and the approach to each patient must be individualised. In this patient population the severity of comorbid conditions and the functional status are of utmost importance in defining the extent of investigation and the therapeutic goals.

A detailed clinical evaluation is the most important aspect in the assessment of elderly patients with LUTS. It has to characterise the voiding symptoms as well as the patient's general medical condition and mental status, enabling the clinician to make a presumptive diagnosis and identify potentially reversible pathologic conditions.

A careful search for treatable causes of voiding problems that are unrelated to a urological aetiology is very important in the evaluation of elderly patients, particularly in those presenting with urinary incontinence. It has been shown that a significant proportion of these patients have transient problems as a cause for their symptoms. These conditions have been included in the mnemonic "DIAPPERS", including Delirium, Infection, Atrophic vaginitis, Pharmaceuticals, Psychological factors, Excess urine output, Restricted mobility, and Stool impaction (Resnick 1984).

The physical examination is an essential part of the evaluation of elderly patients. It can rule out or identify transient causes of voiding dysfunction as well as established urologic diseases and also evaluate comorbid diseases and the functional ability. In women, the pelvic examination evaluates the existence of genital prolapse as well as atrophic vaginitis or urethritis. It is also important to determine the presence and severity of urinary incontinence with provocative stress testing, although this is not a highly sensitive and specific test for the diagnosis of genuine stress incontinence (Cundiff et al. 1997). The rectal examination is important to detect prostate diseases in men and stool impaction and the integrity of sacral innervation in both men and women. The presence of an enlarged prostate on rectal examination is consistent with bladder outlet obstruction and may warrant further investigation. However, it does not confirm or rule out BPH as the cause of prostate enlargement nor does it confirm the existence of bladder outlet obstruction (Gomes et al. 2001).

A minimum urological workup is necessary in every patient presenting with LUTS, including urinalysis, urine culture, pertinent blood tests and PVR measurement. Ideally, a voiding diary of two to three days should be completed by the patient or caregiver to help characterise the patient's usual fluid intake, voiding habits, and severity of incontinence. Radiological evaluation and cystoscopy may be necessary in some patients, particularly if hematuria is present.

3.   Urodynamics

Urodynamics is the dynamic study of transport, storage, and evacuation of urine by the urinary tract. It encompasses various diagnostic tests, including uroflowmetry, cystometry, urethral pressure profile, pressure-flow studies, electromyography of the pelvic floor, and simultaneous radiographic visualisation of the lower urinary tract (videourodynamics). These tests can be used alone or in combination to evaluate lower urinary tract function. Urodynamic studies are considered a highly valuable tool for the evaluation of patients with lower urinary tract symptoms and most experts agree that they provide the most accurate means of diagnosis of voiding problems. However, the indications for and the type of urodynamics necessary for each patient are controversial.

Elderly patients may present with LUTS that are secondary to changes in the lower urinary tract organs that occur with aging and are not pathological conditions. In addition, urinary symptoms in elderly people often have multiple causes because of the higher prevalence of comorbid states such as previous urological surgeries, stroke, dementia, Parkinson's disease, and use of medications. Moreover, some urodynamic findings like detrusor instability and detrusor hyperactivity with impaired contractility are frequent in the geriatric population and may mimic common urological problems such as stress incontinence or outlet obstruction. For these reasons and because the symptoms are poor predictors of urodynamic diagnosis, some authors believe that urodynamic studies should be used liberally in elderly people (Castleden et al. 1981). In general, however, most urologists obtain a urodynamic evaluation only after ruling out reversible causes of voiding dysfunction and when the initial conservative treatment failed to improve the patient's symptoms and/or the clinical assessment did not provide a diagnosis for the voiding problems. The authors believe urodynamics should always be performed in elderly patients with significant lower urinary tract symptoms and coexisting neurological disease, previous surgery on the lower urinary tract, high post-void residual volumes, and whenever a surgical procedure is being considered.

Although urodynamics is an important part of the clinical evaluation of a patient, it has to be analysed in conjunction with all other information obtained from history and physical examination, voiding diaries, as well as radiographic and endoscopic exams. Ultimately, it is essential that urodynamic studies reproduce the patient's symptoms during the test to assure the validity of the urodynamic findings. This is not always easy for numerous reasons, particularly in elderly people. First, the test is performed in an unfriendly environment that includes the presence of the examiner and staff as well as the equipment. Moreover, the introduction of one or two catheters transurethrally in the bladder and another catheter in the rectum can be quite uncomfortable. Finally, a number of potential pitfalls may occur in a urodynamic study, relating to fluid fill rate and temperature, patient position, catheter size, and presence of significant genital prolapse. Despite all of these factors, it has been shown that urodynamics is safe and reliable in the elderly population (Griffiths et al. 1992, Tammela et al. 1999).

3.1   Uroflowmetry

Uroflowmetry is the measurement of urine flow over time and is an important test for the evaluation of the voiding phase of the micturition cycle. It is a simple, objective, and non-invasive urodynamic study that may demonstrate an abnormal urinary pattern and can be used to identify patients who may need a more complex urodynamic test. As the urinary flow is a function of both detrusor contractility and bladder outlet resistance (BOO), it does not establish a definite diagnosis. A normal flow rate can be present in a patient with significant infravesical obstruction, as long as the detrusor can compensate for the increased urethral resistance. Likewise, a weak urinary stream can be seen in a patient with severe outlet obstruction but also in a female patient with detrusor failure.

The single most important parameter of the uroflowmetry is the peak urinary flow (Q_{max}), which is volume dependent (Drach et al. 1979). In general, a $Q_{max} < -15$ ml/s with a voided volume of at least 150 ml is considered low, and may indicate either detrusor hypocontractility or BOO (Fig. 1). The distinction between the two conditions can only be made through pressure-flow studies. The flow rate may be potentially affected by the voided volume, type of flowmeter, and abdominal straining, and it has intrapatient variations. In elderly people, an adequate uroflow measurement may be difficult to obtain. Reasons for that include: (1) geriatric patients commonly void small volumes; (2) the bladder may be empty at the moment of the study and the patient may have urgency or urge-incontinence; (3) mental status may be limiting, and (4) some patients have difficulty voiding in an unfriendly/unfamiliar place.

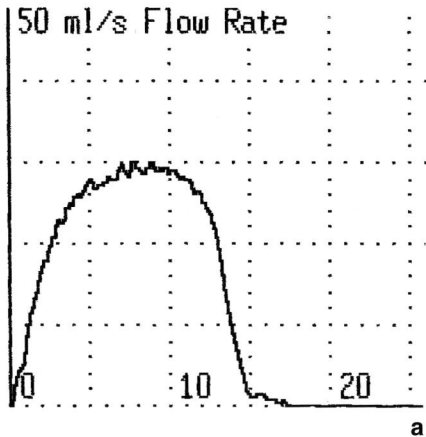

a

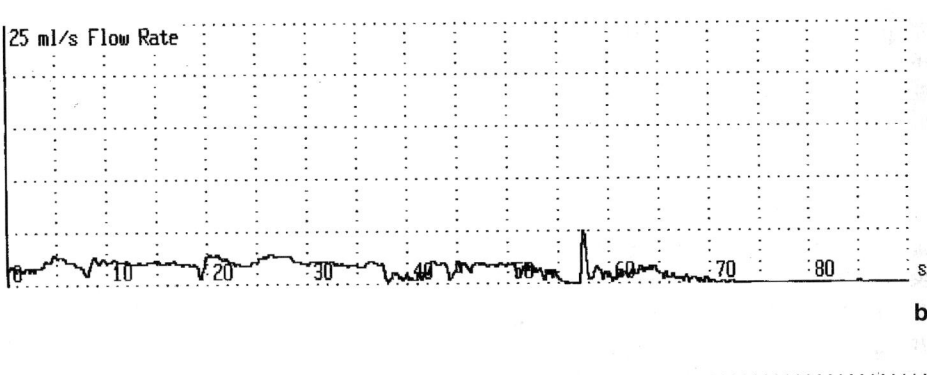

b

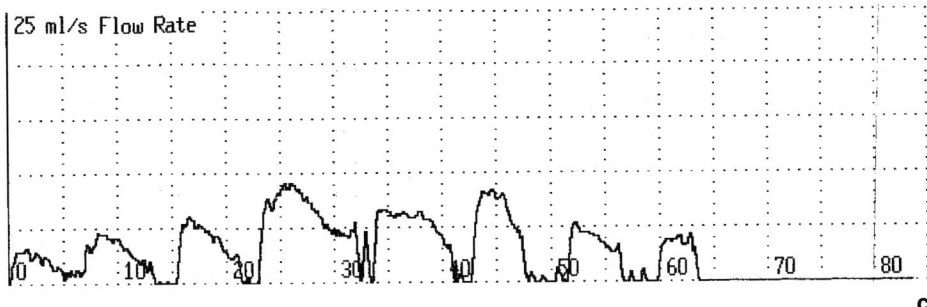

c

Fig. 1. Uroflowmetry. **a** Normal uroflow ($Q_{max} = 30$ ml/s) in a 67-year-old man 6 months after a transurethral resection of the prostate presenting with irritative symptoms. His cystometrogram and pressure-flow studies are shown on Figs. 2a and 3a, respectively; **b** Obstructive uroflow in a 75-year-old man with severe voiding symptoms. The flow pattern shows a sustained low flow rate that is consistent with but not diagnostic of bladder obstruction. Follow-up pressure-flow study confirmed severe bladder obstruction (Fig. 3b); **c** Interrupted uroflow due to abdominal straining in an 80-year-old diabetic man presenting with urge-incontinence and obstructive symptoms and a high postvoid residual (300 ml). Follow-up pressure-flow study confirmed detrusor hyperactivity and impaired contractility (Fig. 2b)

Despite its limitations in diagnosing BOO, uroflowmetry is a sensitive indicator of voiding dysfunction and can be used to distinguish patients who will promptly need further investigation from those that can be started on a treatment regimen and avoid extensive urodynamic testing. It can also be used in patients with known BOO as a measure of progression of the disease or to determine the efficacy of treatment modalities that are expected to improve bladder emptying.

3.2   Residual urine measurement

The post-void residual urine (PVR) is the total volume of urine remaining in the bladder after voiding. It should be measured after an intentional void since an incontinent patient may be able to partially suppress an involuntary detrusor contraction and the PVR will be overestimated. It can be accurately measured with a bladder catheter or by ultrasound and has a significant intraindividual variability in elderly patients (Griffiths et al. 1996). Despite the fact that it does not correlate well with signs and symptoms of bladder obstruction and the inherent variability of the measurement, the PVR is an important part of the clinical investigation of elderly men and women. As the urinary flow, the PVR is a function of both detrusor contractility and bladder outlet resistance (BOO), and does not establish a definite diagnosis of obstruction or detrusor hypocontractility. However, it can be used to identify patients at risk for these conditions as well as to monitor the progression of the disease in patients with known BOO. In general, a PVR of >100 ml is considered high in a male elderly patient. Female patients tend to have lower PVR volumes than male patients (Bonde et al. 1996, Griffiths et al. 1996).

3.3   Cystometry

Cystometry is a measure of the bladder's response to filling and evaluates the filling/reservoir phase of micturition. Many variables should be studied during cystometry, including the bladder capacity, sensation, compliance, presence of involuntary detrusor contractions, and ability of the urethral sphincter to resist increases in abdominal pressure. Although it can be performed with different methods and technical variations, our review will present cystometry as a multichannel study, monitoring both vesical and abdominal pressure and allowing for automatic calculation of the detrusor pressure. However, since urodynamic setups are not available in many geriatric facilities, some authors have proposed a simple bedside evaluation by using a urethral catheter connected to a 50 ml syringe that is used to fill the bladder under gravity. This method also called eyeball urodynamics, may provide useful information on the bladder behaviour during filling, but has obvious limitations compared with standard urodynamics.

As noted before, many aspects of the physiology of micturition may change as part of normal aging and may or may not play a pathogenic role in voiding dysfunction. A very common urodynamic finding in elderly patients is detrusor instability (DI), which is a major cause of urinary incontinence in elderly men and women (Fig. 2a) (Payne 1998, Hampel et al. 1997). However, DI can also be observed in asymptomatic elderly patients, occurring in up to 50% of these subjects (Andersen et al. 1978). This fact emphasizes the importance of reproducing the patient's symptoms during the urodynamic test and also to analyse its results in conjunction with all other information obtained from history and physical examination as well as other exams.

DI in the geriatric population may be associated with impaired detrusor contractility, even in the absence of bladder obstruction. This condition, known as detrusor hyperactivity with impaired contractile function (DHIC),

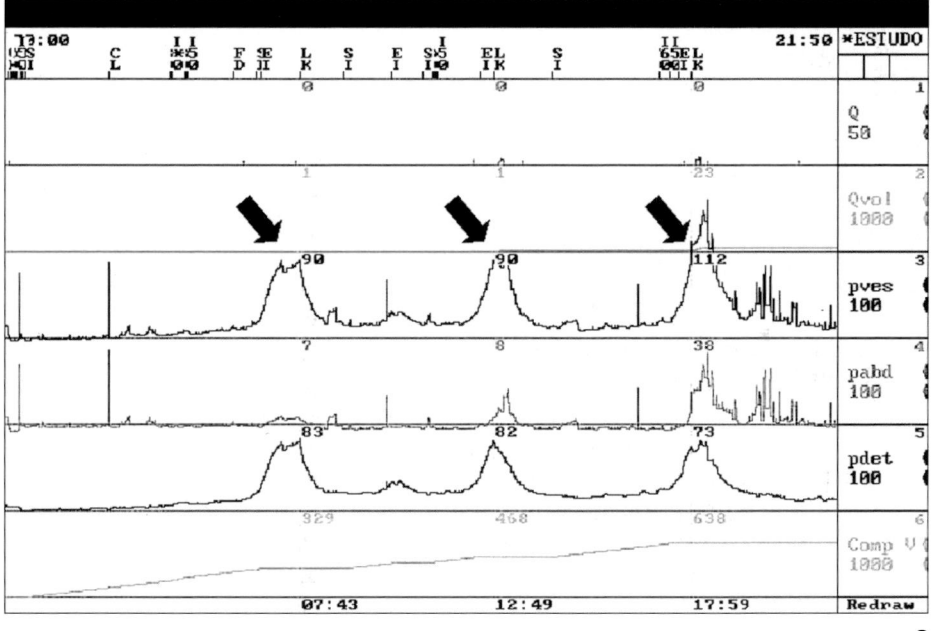

a

Fig. 2. Cystometric findings in the elderly. **a** Multichannel urodynamics tracing of a 67-year-old men complaining of frequency, urgency and urge-incontinence 6 months after transurethral resection of the prostate showing three episodes of detrusor instability accompanied by urge-incontinence (arrows). His voiding study showed complete emptying with a high flow and low detrusor pressure (Fig. 3a). The patient was started on anticholinergic medication and bladder training with great clinical improvement; **b** An 80-year-old man complaining of the same symptoms of the previous patient. His pressure-flow study shows multiple low pressure involuntary detrusor contractions during filling (arrow heads) and a low flow rate associated with abdominal straining and no detectable detrusor contraction in the voiding phase (arrows). Anticholinergic medications should be used cautiously in this patient because of the risk of precipitating urinary retention

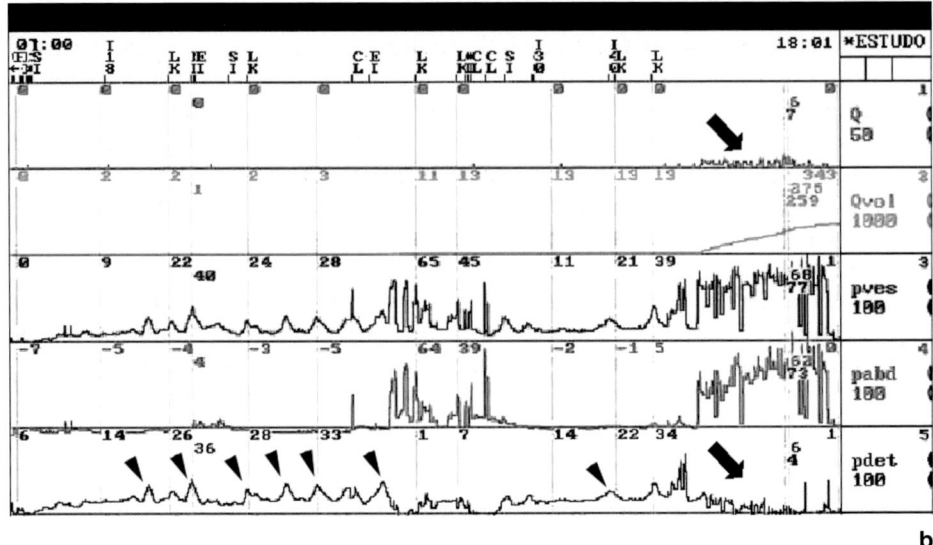

Fig. 2. (continued)

was described by Resnick and Yalla (Resnick and Yalla 1987) and may be a challenging cause of LUTS (Fig. 2b). The pathogenic process that leads to DHIC is unknown (Griffiths et al. 2002). Clinically, patients with DHIC may be no different from patients with DI and normal contractility. In the urodynamics, patients with DHIC have higher post-void residual urine and are not capable to generate effective detrusor contractions in the voiding phase of the study. No signs of bladder obstruction or sphincteric abnormalities are found in their urodynamic tests. The clinical implications associated with the diagnosis of DHIC are very important and emphasise the importance of performing urodynamic studies in elderly patients with voiding dysfunction. DHIC must be distinguished from bladder outlet obstruction, which can also lead to high PVR and may be accompanied by DI in up to 50% of the patients (Gomes et al. 2001). The treatment for the latter may involve α-blocking agents or surgical desobtruction while patients with DHIC have a limited range of therapeutical options. DHIC can mimic a number of other clinical conditions, including urge and stress incontinence and sensory urgency. Again, the appropriate urodynamic diagnosis is very important to enable counselling and a better treatment selection. Patients with urge-incontinence and normal detrusor contractility can be treated safely with bladder training and anticholinergic medications, while patients with DHIC are at high risk for developing urinary retention when they take anticholinergic drugs.

Stress incontinence is an important cause of urinary incontinence in elderly women and may be associated with urge incontinence (mixed urinary incontinence) (Hampel et al. 1997, Payne 1998). In the male population, stress incontinence is uncommon and usually secondary to prostate surgery and/or pelvic radiation or trauma. Elderly patients with suspected stress urinary incontinence should be tested with standard determination of the abdominal (or Valsalva) leak point pressure to determine the magnitude of urethral sphincter damage. The technique for this is the same as in younger adults but special attention must be paid to assure that the test is performed with a relaxed bladder (no detrusor activity during the stress manoeuvres) and also to distinguish between stress incontinence and stress-induced detrusor instability, which can mimic genuine stress incontinence (McGuire et al. 1996). The results of the abdominal leak point pressure test may be important in selecting appropriate treatment, since it has been shown that patients with significant intrinsic sphincter deficiency are not good candidates for pelvic floor rehabilitation and also have poor results after bladder neck suspension procedures. These patients may be better treated by a sling procedure or an injectable agent (McGuire et al. 1996).

3.4   Pressure-flow studies of micturition

Disorders of the voiding phase of the micturition cycle are very common in elderly patients. As noted before, measurement of the urinary flow rate and post-void residual volume can indicate the existence of an abnormality and even suggest a possible aetiology for the problem, but its exact nature and severity can only be determined by using a more complex urodynamic test that simultaneously measures the uroflow and detrusor pressure. This test, known as pressure-flow study, enables the analysis of detrusor contractility and bladder outlet resistance (obstruction). Unless the patient has a significant functional disability or cognitive impairment, it is a simple test to perform in most patients being submitted to a cystometry, since the only technical difference is that a uroflowmetry is added to the study and the patient is required to void when his/her bladder is full.

Pressure-flow studies identify three fundamental voiding states: (1) low detrusor pressure with normal flow (unobstructed); (2) high detrusor pressure with low flow (obstructed), and (3) low detrusor pressure with low flow (poor detrusor contractility) (Figs. 2b, 3a and 3b). The importance of establishing these urodynamic diagnoses is obvious, since the prognosis and treatment alternatives for patients presenting with these conditions are completely different. In the elderly population, LUTS suggestive of BOO are commonly caused by pathophysiological conditions other than bladder obstruction, and even women may have obstructive symptoms in the absence of bladder obstruction (Madersbacher et al. 1999b, Griffiths et al. 2002, Madersbacher et al. 1998).

Abnormal voiding can affect the bladder's ability to store and result in an abnormal cystometrogram. Detrusor instability and low bladder compliance are cystometric abnormalities that can be present in a significant number of patients with bladder outlet obstruction (Abrams et al. 1979, Madersbacher et al. 1999a, Rosier et al. 1995). They may improve in many patients after the relief of obstruction but in the geriatric population detrusor instability and urge incontinence may be the result of age-associated changes and not secondary to obstruction (Madersbacher et al. 1999a, Abrams et al. 1979). As a result, elderly patients who are potential candidates for prostatic surgery may have a worse prognosis, and detrusor instability is likely to persist following surgery to relieve BOO (Gormley et al. 1993). This is also true for elderly patients with neurological diseases such as Parkinson disease, cerebrovascular accident, and multiple sclerosis, who are at high risk of having a poor outcome after a prostate surgery and should be investigated with complete urodynamic studies before a decision is made to operate on these patients (Cockett et al. 1993).

Bladder outlet obstruction is an uncommon diagnosis in women. When present, this condition may be secondary to an anti-incontinence procedure severe genital prolapse or dysfunctional voiding (Nitti et al. 1999). It is well known, however, that aging women may report voiding symptoms similar to age matched men despite the fact that they do not have prostate-related

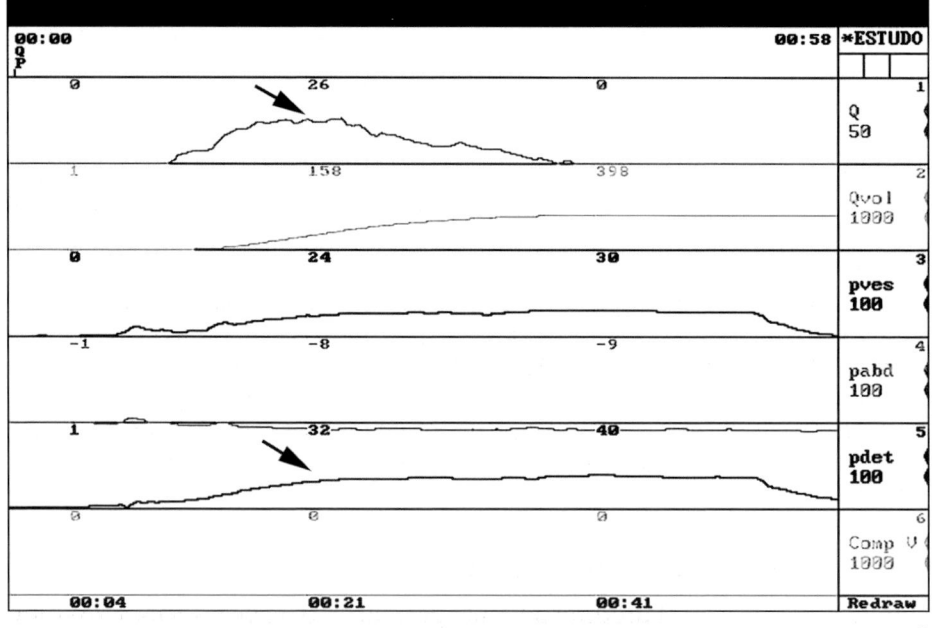

a

Fig. 3. Pressure-flow studies of micturition. **a** Voiding study of a 67-year-old men with unobstructed flow 6 months after transurethral resection of the prostate (cystometry showed on Fig. 2a). The urodynamic tracings show a good maximum flow rate ($Q_{max} = 26$ ml/s – superior arrow) and a corresponding low detrusor pressure ($P_{detQmax} = 32$ cm H_2O – inferior arrow); **b** A 75-year-old man with a history of severe obstructive symptoms of decreased flow and hesitancy. His urodynamic study shows a high pressure-low flow pattern configuring bladder outlet obstruction ($Q_{max} = 4$ ml/s – superior arrow and $P_{detQmax} = 168$ cm H_2O – inferior arrow). The patient was treated with a transurethral resection of the prostate

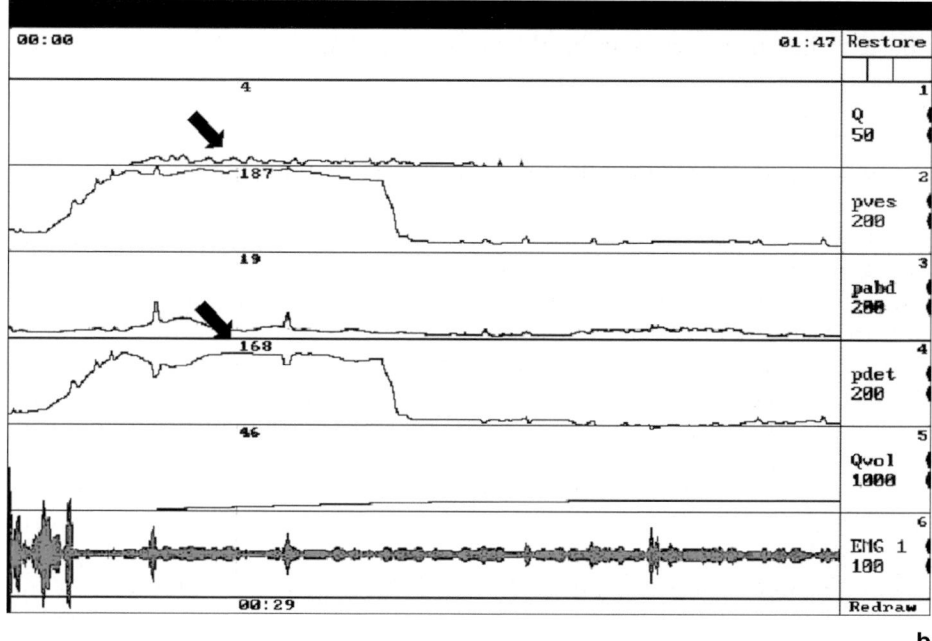

Fig. 3. *(continued)*

voiding problems. Madersbacher et al. have compared age-related changes of urodynamic parameters in both sexes and shown that age-associated urodynamic changes in both sexes are comparable for a number of parameters, including increase of post-void residual volume and a decrease of peak flow rate, voided volume and bladder capacity (Madersbacher et al. 1998). With respect to detrusor instability, they observed an increase in men from 23.4% (40–60 years) to 46.7% (>80 years), whereas in women no significant age-related changes were present. These findings provide an explanation for the fact that aging women report comparable voiding symptoms as men and suggest a primary, non-sex-specific aging process of the urinary bladder.

3.5   Urethral pressure profile (UPP)

Different techniques of urethral pressure profilometry have been used to study sphincteric function in patients with urinary incontinence and to evaluate patients with suspected obstruction (Constantinou and Christensen 1996, Sullivan et al. 1996). However, the value of UPP in these clinical settings is controversial. The correlation between UPP measurements and the presence of incontinence or continence in a number of clinical situations is poor (Nager et al. 2001). Low urethral pressures, predicting incontinence, have been found in continent elderly patients (Diokno et al. 1990). The authors do not routinely use UPP in the evaluation of patients with LUTS. Measurement of the leak point pressures has been shown to be a more reliable method of assessing sphincteric function and is also more practical since it is a part of the filling phase of the study (cystometry) (McGuire et al. 1996).

3.6 Videourodynamics

Videourodynamic studies consist of using a radiopaque contrast filling medium for urodynamics to allow simultaneous fluoroscopic visualisation of the bladder and urethra during the filling and emptying phases. This technique is considered the most complete and precise urodynamic test, since it allows simultaneous pressure measurements with structural information (Fig. 4). Despite the advantages of having anatomical information associated with the functional data, the indications for videourodynamics are not very clear. The study requires a more expensive and complex equipment that is not available at many urological facilities. Moreover, it uses radiation, with its attendant problems and risks. In addition, it has not been shown that videourodynamics are superior to standard urodynamics in most clinical settings. For these reasons, most urologists perform videourodynamics only in the more complex cases involving suspected anatomic abnormalities, failure of previous surgical procedures or associated neurological problems.

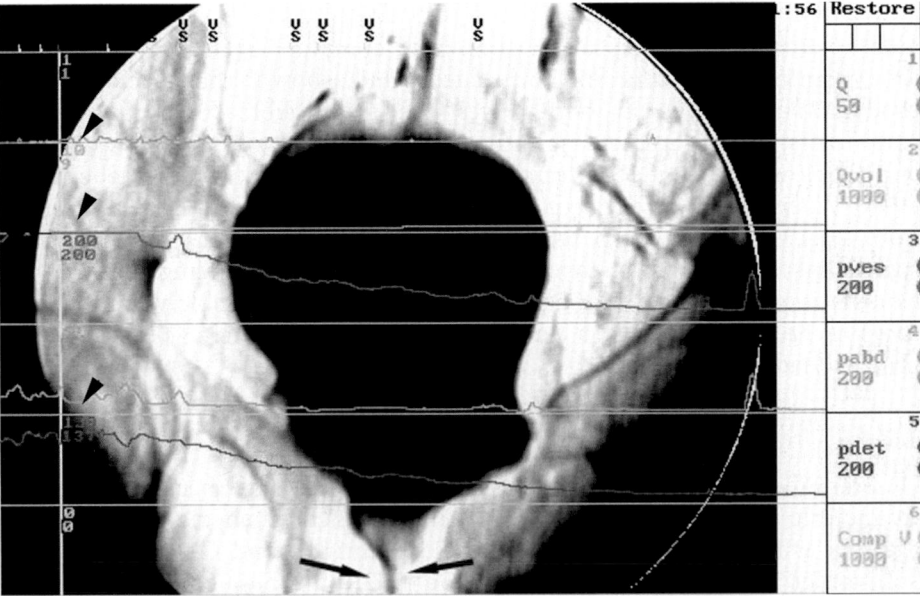

Fig. 4. Videourodynamics. A 64-year-old woman complaining of hesitancy, low flow and frequency 2 years after a transvaginal anti-incontinence surgery and 1 year after a cerebrovascular accident. The voiding study demonstrates a high pressure-low flow pattern (arrow heads) and the level of obstruction is shown at the midurethra (arrows). The patient was submitted to a urethrolysis procedure with great improvement of the obstructive symptoms

4.   Closing remarks

Urodynamics is a highly valuable and safe tool in the investigation of elderly patients with LUTS with or without incontinence. Incontinence and other LUTS may be a manifestation of a subacute or reversible process within or outside of the lower urinary tract, and may be effectively treated in most instances. Urodynamics is not always necessary and should be indicated after excluding potentially reversible conditions outside the urinary tract that may be causing or contributing to the symptoms. The initial evaluation of an incontinent geriatric patient includes a targeted history and physical examination, urinalysis, voiding diaries and simple tests of lower urinary tract function like uroflowmetry and PVR. This evaluation should allow the clinician to identify patients who will need more complex urodynamic tests including those for whom a presumptive diagnosis cannot be made and those that failed initial conservative treatment.

Urodynamic findings in elderly patients may include common diagnoses such as bladder outlet obstruction and stress urinary incontinence. However, urological problems often coexist in elderly patients, and conditions such as detrusor instability and impaired detrusor contractility are common. The identification of these conditions is necessary to assure accurate prognostic counselling and treatment selection.

5.   References

1. Abrams PH, Farrar DJ, Turner WR, Whiteside CG, Feneley RC (1979) The results of prostatectomy: a symptomatic and urodynamic analysis of 152 patients. J Urol 121: 640–642
2. Andersen JT, Jacobsen O, Worm-Petersen J, Hald T (1978) Bladder function in healthy elderly males. Scand J Urol Nephrol 12: 123–127
3. Bonde HV, Sejr T, Erdmann L, Meyhoff HH, Lendorf A, Rosenkilde P, Bodker A, Nielsen MB (1996) Residual urine in 75-year-old men and women. A normative population study. Scand J Urol Nephrol 30: 89–91
4. Boone TB (1996a) Urodynamics I. Urol Clin North Am 23: 171–336
5. Boone TB (1996b) Urodynamics II. Urol Clin North Am 23: 337–520
6. Castleden CM, Duffin HM, Asher MJ (1981) Clinical and urodynamic studies in 100 elderly incontinent patients. Br Med J (Clin Res Ed) 282: 1103–1105
7. Chiarelli P, Brown WJ (1999) Leaking urine in Australian women: prevalence and associated conditions. Women Health 29: 1–13
8. Cockett AT, Khoury S, Aso Y (1993) Proceedings of the 2nd International Consultation on Benign Prostatic Hyperplasia (BPH). Scientific Communications International Ltd: Jersey
9. Constantinou CE, Christensen LL (1996) Urethral pressures in the study of female incontinence. In: Raz S (ed) Female urology. W.B. Saunders: Philadelphia, pp 115–131
10. Cundiff GW, Harris RL, Coates KW, Bump RC (1997) Clinical predictors of urinary incontinence in women. Am J Obstet Gynecol 177: 262–266
11. Damian J, Martin-Moreno JM, Lobo F, Bonache J, Cervino J, Redondo-Marquez L, Martinez-Agullo E (1998) Prevalence of urinary incontinence among Spanish older people living at home. Eur Urol 34: 333–338

12. Diokno AC, Normolle DP, Brown MB, Herzog AR (1990) Urodynamic tests for female geriatric urinary incontinence. Urology 36: 431–439
13. Drach GW, Layton TN, Binard WJ (1979) Male peak urinary flow rate: relationships to volume voided and age. J Urol 122: 210–214
14. Fantl JA, Newman DK, Colling J, DeLancey JO, Keeys C, Loughery R, McDowell BJ, Norton P, Ouslander J, Schnelle J, Staskin D, Tries J, Urich V, Whitmore KE, Weiss BD, Whitmore KE (1996) Urinary incontinence in adults: Acute and chronic management. Clinical Practice Guideline 2. Rockville, MD: U.S. Department of Health and Human Services. Clinical Practice Guidelines, Public Health Service, Agency for Health Care Policy and Research
15. Gomes CM, Trigo-Rocha F, Arap MA, Arap S (2001) Bladder outlet obstruction and urodynamic evaluation in patients with benign prostatic hyperplasia. Braz J Urol 27: 575–588
16. Gormley EA, Griffiths DJ, McCracken PN, Harrison GM, McPhee MS (1993) Effect of transurethral resection of the prostate on detrusor instability and urge incontinence in elderly males. Neurourol Urodyn 12: 445–453
17. Griffiths DJ, Harrison G, Moore K, McCracken P (1996) Variability of post-void residual urine volume in the elderly. Urol Res 24: 23–26
18. Griffiths DJ, McCracken PN, Harrison GM, Gormley EA (1992) Characteristics of urinary incontinence in elderly patients studied by 24-hour monitoring and urodynamic testing. Age Aging 21: 195–201
19. Griffiths DJ, McCracken PN, Harrison GM, Gormley EA, Moore KN (2002) Urge incontinence and impaired detrusor contractility in the elderly. Neurourol Urodyn 21: 126–131
20. Haidinger G, Madersbacher S, Waldhoer T, Lunglmayr G, Vutuc C (1999) The prevalence of lower urinary tract symptoms in Austrian males and associations with sociodemographic variables. Eur J Epidemiol 15: 717–722
21. Hampel C, Wienhold D, Benken C, Eggersmann C, Thüroff JW (1997) Definition of overactive bladder and epidemiology of urinary incontinence. Urology 50: 4–14
22. Homma Y, Imajo C, Takahashi S, Kawabe K, Aso Y (1994) Urinary symptoms and urodynamics in a normal elderly population. Scand J Urol Nephrol 157 [Suppl]: 27–30
23. Koskimaki J, Hakama M, Huhtala H, Tammela TL (1998) Prevalence of lower urinary tract symptoms in Finnish men: a population- based study. Br J Urol 81: 364–369
24. Madersbacher S, Pycha A, Klingler CH, Mian C, Djavan B, Stulnig T, Marberger M (1999a) Interrelationships of bladder compliance with age, detrusor instability, and obstruction in elderly men with lower urinary tract symptoms. Neurourol Urodyn 18: 3–15
25. Madersbacher S, Pycha A, Klingler CH, Schatzl G, Marberger M (1999b) The International Prostate Symptom score in both sexes: a urodynamics-based comparison. Neurourol Urodyn 18: 173–182
26. Madersbacher S, Pycha A, Schatzl G, Mian C, Klingler CH, Marberger M (1998) The aging lower urinary tract: a comparative urodynamic study of men and women. Urology 51: 206–212
27. McGuire EJ, Ccspcdcs RD, O'Connell HE (1996) Leak-point pressures. Urol Clin North Am 23: 253–262
28. Mundy AR, Stephenson TP, Wein AJ (1994) Urodynamics: principles, practice and application. Churchill Livingstone, Edinburgh

29. Nager CW, Schulz JA, Stanton SL, Monga A (2001) Correlation of urethral closure pressure, leak-point pressure and incontinence severity measures. Int Urogynecol J Pelvic Floor Dysfunct 12: 395–400
30. Nitti VW (1998) Practical urodynamics. W.B. Saunders Company: Philadelphia, Pennsylvania
31. Nitti VW, Tu LM, Gitlin J (1999) Diagnosing bladder outlet obstruction in women. J Urol 161: 1535–1540
32. Payne CK (1998) Epidemiology, pathophysiology, and evaluation of urinary incontinence and overactive bladder. Urology 51: 3–10
33. Resnick NM (1984) Urinary incontinence in the elderly. Med Grand Rounds 3: 281–290
34. Resnick NM, Elbadawi A, Yalla SV (1995) Age and the lower urinary tract: What is normal? Neurourol Urodyn 14: 577–579
35. Resnick NM, Yalla SV (1987) Detrusor hyperactivity with impaired contractile function. An unrecognized but common cause of incontinence in elderly patients. JAMA 257: 3076–3081
36. Roberts RO, Jacobsen SJ, Rhodes T, Reilly WT, Girman CJ, Talley NJ, Lieber MM (1998) Urinary incontinence in a community-based cohort: prevalence and healthcare-seeking. J Am Geriatr Soc 46: 467–472
37. Rosier PF, de la Rosette JJ, Wijkstra H, van Kerrebroeck PE, Debruyne FM (1995) Is detrusor instability in elderly males related to the grade of obstruction? Neurourol Urodyn 14: 625–633
38. Rovner ES, Gomes CM, Trigo-Rocha F, Arap S, Wein AJ (2002) Evaluation and treatment of the overactive bladder. Rev Hosp Clin 57: 39–48
39. Schmidbauer J, Temml C, Schatzl G, Haidinger G, Madersbacher S (2001) Risk factors for urinary incontinence in both sexes. Analysis of a health screening project. Eur Urol 39: 565–570
40. Sullivan MP, Comiter CV, Yalla SV (1996) Micturitional urethral pressure profilometry. Urol Clin North Am 23: 263–278
41. Tammela TL, Schäfer W, Barrett DM, Abrams P, Hedlund H, Rollema HJ, Matos FA, Nordling J, Bruskewitz R, Miller P, Kirby R, Andersen JT, Jacobsen C, Gormley GJ, Malice MP, Bach MA (1999) Repeated pressure-flow studies in the evaluation of bladder outlet obstruction due to benign prostatic enlargement. Finasteride Urodynamics Study Group. Neurourol Urodyn 18: 17–24

Correspondence address: Flavio Trigo Rocha, M.D., Head-Section of Urodynamics, Division of Urology, University of São Paulo School of Medicine, Rua Barata Ribeiro, 237 cjs. 104–106, 01308-000 São Paulo, Brazil (E-mail: flaviotrigo@uol.com.br).

Pathophysiology orientated therapy of the aging bladder

C. Hampel[1], *E. Plas*[2], *L. K. Daha*[2], and *J. W. Thüroff*[1]

[1]Department of Urology, Johannes Gutenberg University Mainz, Germany
[2]Department of Urology and LBI for Urology & Andrology,
Lainz Hospital, Vienna, Austria

Contents

1.   Introduction

Aging is associated with changes of organ systems including skin, bone metabolism and the muscoloskeletal, endocrine, cardiovascular, and genitourinary systems. Concerning age-related changes in lower urinary tract function, the incidence of nocturia and general neurological or vascular diseases with impact on detrusor function are comparable for men and women. However, there are also sex related differences in lower urinary tract symptoms (LUTS) such as bladder outlet obstruction in men (due to age-related prostate growth) and gonadal insufficiency, multiparity, cystocele or enterocele in women. In addition to the common occurrence of LUTS in elderly people, comorbidity increases with age, often resulting in an accumulation of orthopaedic, cardiovascular, endocrine, and urinary tract problems that notably affect quality of life in elderly people.

Affection of detrusor function can be caused by altering the storage or emptying phase of the bladder. Bladder storage problems can be subclassified according to their pathogenesis as hypersensitivity, neurological or idio-pathic hyperactivity, or low compliance bladder. Diagnosis is confirmed by urodynamic studies. Chronic alterations of the detrusor due to fistulas, irradiation, pelvic surgery, or interstitial cystitis induce development of low compliance bladder with its associated voiding problems.

Alterations of bladder emptying in the aging process may be related to detrusor function or outlet obstruction. Neurogenic or non neurogenic detrusor hypoactivity and/or bladder outlet obstruction can cause decompensation of the detrusor, resulting in myogenic alteration. Usually, bladder outlet obstruction (BOO) has a morphologic correlate due to prostate enlargement. However, functional obstruction may be caused by neurological affection with consecutive detrusor-sphincter dyssynergia.

Morphological investigations by Elabadawi et al. clearly showed physiological changes of the detrusor correlating with the aging process, such as degeneration of the smooth muscle cells, enlargement and fibrosis of the interstitium, and reduction of nerve endings in the detrusor (Elbadawi et al. 1997a, b; Elbadawi et al. 1993a–d; Hailemariam et al. 1997). In addition to these morphological local changes, reduction of inhibitory central stimuli, bladder or uterine descensus, prolapse, and side effects of pharmaceuticals finally result in a significant alteration of bladder function in elderly people.

Examples for reduction of central inhibition of the detrusor due to neurological disease are Parkinson's disease, apoplexy, and small vessel disease. The reduced inhibition of peripheral reflex bounds via the pontine micturition centre lead to an uninhibited urinary bladder with detrusor hyperactivity.

One of the problems in the aging detrusor is the lack of data concerning definition of a normal bladder function in elderly people, but comprehensively it may be suggested that the normal aging bladder is characterised by detrusor stability, lack of obstruction, and normal contractility. Although bladder function can remain normal during aging, ultrastructural alterations of the detrusor occur – so called dense-band patterns of the detrusor. Smooth muscle cells are compacted with normal structure, but a reduction in superficial membrane vesicles occur that may be related to a reduction in cellular calcium exchange or with storage of neurotransmitters.

As shown above, the aging detrusor is characterised by three different complexes:

1. Hyperactivity
2. Hypocontractility
3. Obstruction.

Although an interaction exists between all three mechanisms, one should analyse each factor with its possible influence on the aging detrusor.

2. Therapeutic options of the aging bladder

2.1 Detrusor hyperactivity

Hyperactivity is the predominant problem in elderly people, affecting the filling phase with its symptoms of pollakisuria, nocturia, urgency, and urge incontinence as often found in urodynamic studies (Fig. 1). Elbadawi was the first investigator reporting on the correlation of ultrastructural detrusor changes and urodynamics. In patients with detrusor hyperactivity without outlet obstruction, a disjunction pattern of the bladder detrusor was reported in between neighbouring smooth muscle cells and an enlarged

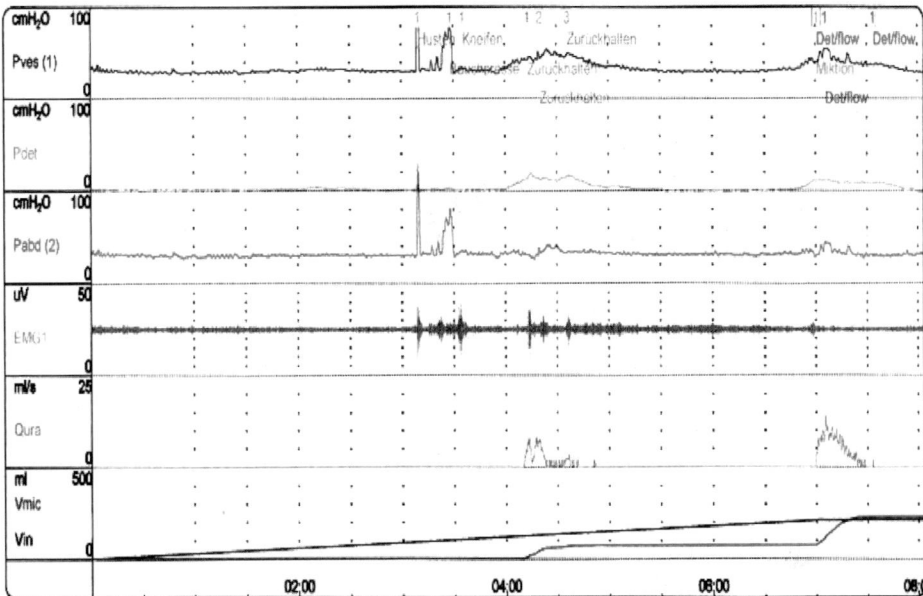

Fig. 1. Characteristic urodynamic study of a patient with urge incontinence – uninhibited detrusor contractions cause urinary leakage in the absence of involuntary urine loss during abdominal exercise (coughing and valsalva manoeuvre), the functional bladder capacity is small, although the compliance of the detrusor is normal (>25 ml/cm H_2O)

interstitium. These changes may be related to alterations in electrical signalling in the detrusor, which may cause hyperactivity.

Hyperactivity is the contraction of the detrusor without permission, as stated by McGuire. If hyperactivity of the detrusor is found, it should be differentiated into its idiopathic form or secondary to obstruction or neurological disorders. However, detrusor hyperactivity was found in asymptomatic volunteer women in up to 68% in ambulatory monitoring (Heslington and Hilton 1996). In case of obstruction, deobstruction will often relieve symptoms and causally treat dysfunction, but in case of idiopathic or neurogenic hyperactivity, only pharmaceutical and behavioural treatment intervention may improve symptoms.

Antimuscarinic drugs are the substances used most often in the treatment of detrusor hyperactivity. Although several substances are available, some are considered to be of merely historical interest as they have severe side effects. Antimuscarinics are antagonists of acetylcholine at the level of muscarinic receptor binding (M1–M5); 80% of the muscarinic receptors of the bladder are M2 receptors. The remaining 20% are M3 receptors, which are mainly responsible for detrusor contractions by activation of adenosine-tri-phosphate induced liberalisation of calcium, with consecutive muscle contraction. The activation of M2 receptors leads to inhibition of adenylate cyclase, which results in augmentation of cyclic adenosine monophosphate (cAMP) level and bladder relaxation (Hegde and Eglen 1999) (Fig. 2). According to their chemical

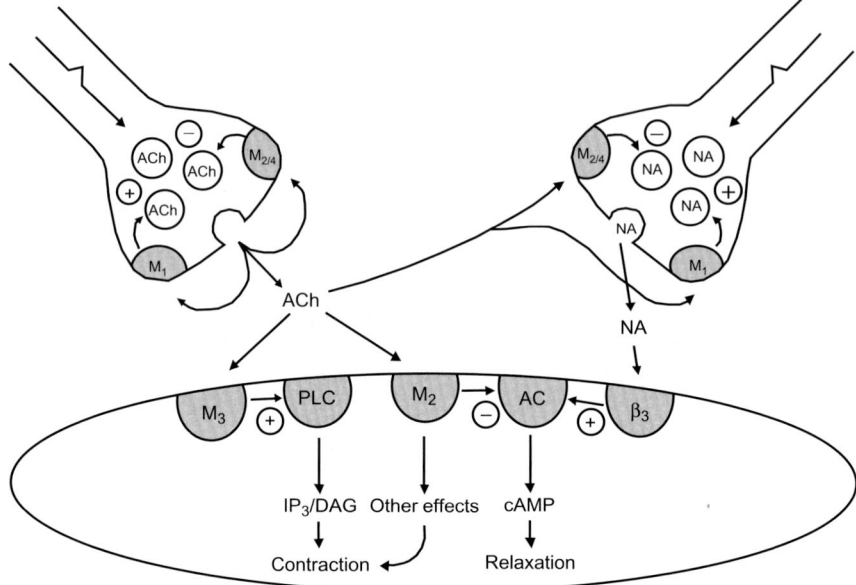

Fig. 2. Pre- and postjunctional muscarinic receptor subtype distribution and subtype specific mode of action in the urinary bladder (*AC* adenylate cyclase; *ACh* acetylcholine; *cAMP* cyclic adenosine monophosphate; *DAG* diacylglycerol; *IP₃* inositol-trisphosphate; *NA* noradrenaline; *PLC* phospholipase C) (Chapple 2000)

structure antimuscarinics can be differentiated into tertiary or quaternary amines. Tertiary amines are resorbed rapidly and nearly completely in the intestine, whereas quaternary amines have a slower absorption time and do not cross the blood-brain barrier. The difference in absorption may be compensated by dose titration of quaternary amines. Several antimuscarinic pharmaceuticals are available, with proved efficacy in all cases (Fig. 3).

Side effects of anticholinergics represent the whole spectrum of systems involved with M1–M5 receptors, such as increase in intraocular pressure, problems with accommodation, dryness of the mouth, constipation, and voiding dysfunction. Central nervous side effects such as impaired concentration occur only in tertiary amines that cross the blood-brain barrier. Due to the drugs' parasympatholytic activity caution is advised in patients with tachycardia or cerebrovascular insufficiency, as symptoms may become aggravated in some cases. Contraindications for antimuscarinics are obstruction of the gastrointestinal tract, achalasia, megacolon, glaucoma, tachyarrhythmia and cardial insufficiency, cerebrovascular insufficiency, and myasthenia gravis. Apart from pharmacokinetic differences of tertiary and quaternary amines, the bioavailability of antimuscarinics can be different due to protein binding. Binding of hormones or pharmaceuticals to proteins is of increasing interest in the aging process as its leads to differences in bioavailability in young and older patients. This may explain differences in the bioavailability of drugs since high protein

		Receptor-Affinity	Side-effects

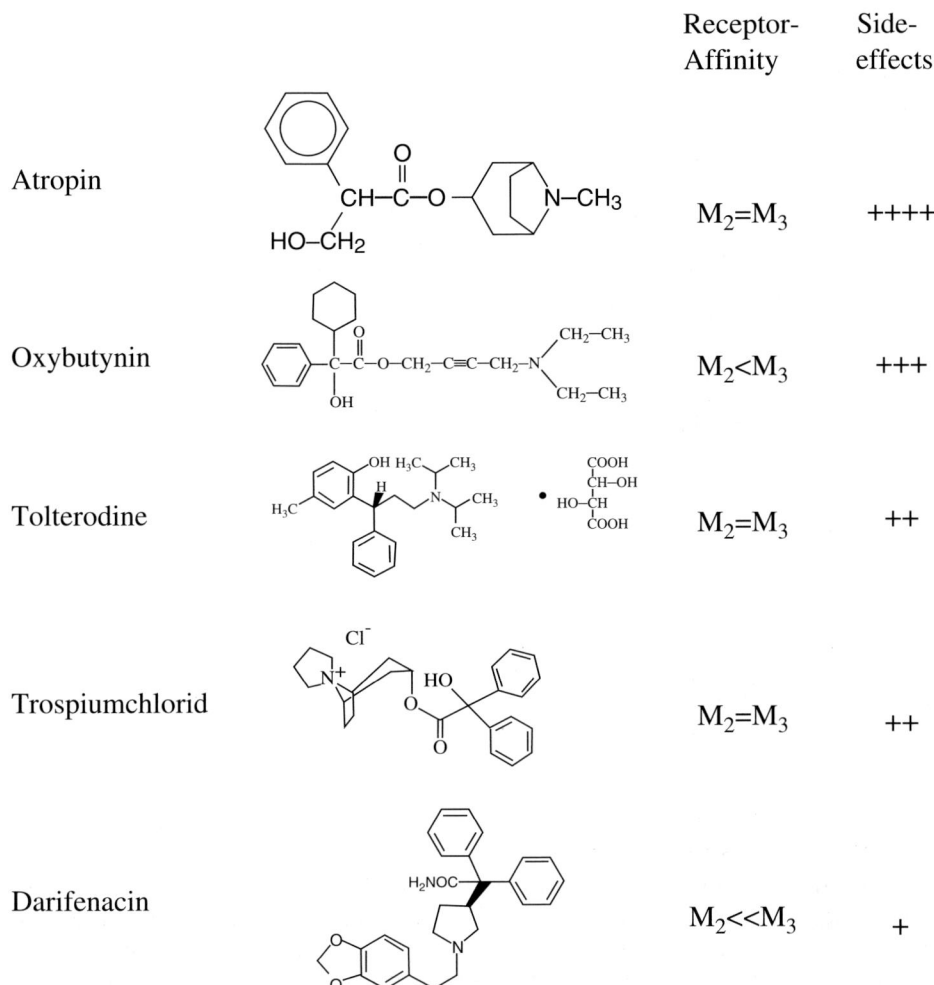

Atropin $\quad M_2=M_3 \quad ++++$

Oxybutynin $\quad M_2<M_3 \quad +++$

Tolterodine $\quad M_2=M_3 \quad ++$

Trospiumchlorid $\quad M_2=M_3 \quad ++$

Darifenacin $\quad M_2<<M_3 \quad +$

Fig. 3. Various antimuscarinics in use for treatment of detrusor hyperactivity

binding does not exclude efficacy of medication. Besides differences in bioavailability half life time vary between $1\frac{1}{2}$ hours and 3 hours. Only propiverin has a longer half life and therefore increases the risk of dose accumulation in elderly patients. Some of the antimuscarinic drugs (oxybutinin, propiverin, trospium) showed an additional analgetic and spasmolytic effect in vitro, but these effects were seen only in higher dosages. Several reports and meta-analysis showed the efficacy of anti-muscarinics in the treatment of bladder hyeractivity. The most well known and commonly used drug, oxybutynin, reduced urgency, pollakisuria and nocturia in patients without obstructions by some 30%, an improvement in urge incontinence was seen in 50%. Randomised trials reported symptom-atic improvement in 74%, associated with a complication rate of 70%

Table 1. Subtype-specific receptor affinity (pKi) of various antimuscarinics in use for treatment of bladder overactivity

	M2 receptor affinity (pKi)	M3 receptor affinity (pKi)
Atropin (Kiwamoto et al. 2001)	9,0	9,4
Propiverin (Kiwamoto et al. 2001)	5,7	6,7
Oxybutynin (Kiwamoto et al. 2001)	7,6	8,7
Tolterodine (Gillberg et al. 1998)	8,4	8,5
Solifenacin (Ikeda et al. 2002)	6,9	8,0
Darifenacin (Gillberg et al. 1998)	7,3	8,9

(Thüroff et al. 1998). Newly developed drugs such as propiverin and tolterodine showed equal efficacy with significantly fewer side effects, although the number of available studies is clearly not as detailed as with oxybutynin. Comparing the severity of side effects of oxybutynin with new available drugs showed that side effects were less common and had only minor severity compared with oxybutynin, which has commonly reported moderate to severe side effects. New agents with major affinity to M3-receptors are darifenacin and solifenacin (Table 1). First results are promising with respect to reduced adverse events with improvement of urgency (Chapple et al. 2002).

Another group of substances that has been used in treating bladder hyperactivity was myotropic spasmolytics such as papaverin and flavoxate. These medications should not be considered as first line medications because of their high dosage requirement and lack of efficacy for detrusor hyperactivity. However, the concept of using muscle relaxants in hyper-active detrusor is still of interest. These drugs block intracellular phos-phodiesterase, an enzyme causing an increase in cyclic AMP, which in turn reduces release of calcium from the sarcoplasmic reticulum. This results in reduction of muscle contractility. Clinical trials studying flavoxate reported a reduction of pollakisuria by 10%, but urge incontinence improved by 50%, with subjective improvement in 44% and side effects of only 25% (Thüroff et al. 1998).

The use of tricyclic antidepressants for bladder hyperactivity relies on different mechanisms, suggesting an anticholinergic, α-adrenergic, and centrally inhibitory effect. Randomised trials showed an improvement in night time incontinence in elderly patients. But side effects increased with dosages (150 mg) required for detrusor hyperactivity improvement. Careful dose titration and avoidance of drug accumulation in aging patients are therefore recommended (Thüroff et al. 1998).

In vitro results of calcium channel blockers indicated clear reduction of detrusor hyperactivity via blocking extracellular to intracellular exchange of calcium. Although clinical trials on flunaricin reported an improvement in symptoms by 78%, the number and severity of side effects were clinically sig-nificant in the dosages required to obtain sufficient clinical improvement.

Another group of substances investigated for detrusor hyperactivity were $\beta2$-adrenergics – especially clenbuterol, which was regularly used by gynaecologists. These drugs inhibit detrusor activity by binding to $\beta2$-detrusor receptors, again activating adenylate cyclase, increasing cAMP, and restricting calcium release. Clinical investigations reported significant subjective improvement in 50%, with side effects in 40% (Thüroff et al. 1998).

In addition to anticholinergics, α-adrenergics, $\beta2$-agonists, calcium channel blockers, amines, and antidepressants, prostaglandin inhibitors such as flurbiprofen have been investigated, both in vitro and in vivo. Although reductions in pollakisuria, nocturia, and urge incontinence were reported by 26%, 48%, and 49% respectively, severe side effects were often reported, which makes these drugs unsuitable for the treatment of detrusor hyperactivity (Palmer 1983).

One important aspect in any randomised placebo controlled trial is the improvement of symptoms in the placebo group. Reviewing all placebo controlled trials showed a reduction in pollakisuria and nocturia in 12% and 13% in the placebo arm. Without the intake of any active compound, urge incontinence was reduced by 22%, with an 37% overall subjective improvement. These percentages emphasise the importance of placebo controlled trials, since 1/3 of improvement can be expected in any trial, no matter whether verum or placebo drugs are given. But placebo does not only induce symptomatic improvement, it also causes side effects, which were reported in up to 33% – again, a percentage that may be subtracted from the high percentages in the verum groups concerning detrusor hyperactivity.

Hyperactivity of the detrusor is the predominant problem in elderly patients. Another often observed functional change of the aging bladder is hypocontractility. The ultrastructural correlate to urodynamically reported hypocontractility is the presence of so called degenerative patterns as described by Elbadawi et al. (1998). These histological patterns represent an extracellular located sarcoplasma due to local cell death, causing extrinsic placement of intracellular compartments. Detrusor biopsies commonly showed no increase in collagen fibres. The reason for these often observed changes are not yet clear. It is most likely to be a multifactorial process due to chronic infravesical obstruction, detrusor decompensation, neurogenic disorders, diabetes, postoperatively denervated detrusor after pelvic surgery, or it may be related to voiding habits ("Banker bladder").

2.2   Detrusor hypocontractility

Since detrusor hypocontractility is often associated with infravesical obstruction, reduction of outflow resistance will be the primary treatment of choice. Before any medical treatment regimen is started, a voiding diary in combination with double voiding and reduction in voiding intervals should be mandatory. If no improvement is seen, then medical treatment may be successful in the acute phase such as post partum or post-operatively. It increases detrusor tonus through directly or indirectly acting parasympathomimetics and reduces outflow resistance by the addition of selective $\alpha 1$- or unselective α-blockers. Although the concept of outflow resistance reduction by α-blockers is promising, randomised trials of its efficacy are lacking, with only case reports available. Unfortunately, complete emptying of the bladder without residual urine can be expected only in some cases. If no improvement of residual urine is achievable, clean intermittent catheterisation (CIC) is the most effective way for prevention of long term effects such as chronic cystitis, pyelonephritis, bladder stones, and deterioration of the upper urinary tract.

2.3   Bladder outlet obstruction

As already shown, chronic infravesical obstruction is one major issue especially of the aging male detrusor. Again, ultrastructural and urodynamic studies by Elbadawi revealed a good correlation of high outflow resistance with enlarged detrusor smooth muscle cells and interstitium, reported as "cholangiosis of the bladder" causing reduction of detrusor compliance. However, obstruction and hypocontractility are often associated with hyperactivity, well known as detrusor hyperactivity impaired contractility with or without obstruction (DHIC detrusor).

Several years ago, Abrams investigated the presence of hyperactivity in patients with bladder outlet obstruction (Abrams et al. 1979). They reported detrusor hyperactivity in 2/3 of the cases. Postoperative re-evaluation after performing transurethral prostate resection or suprapubic adenoma enucleation found normal detrusor function in 50% but 33% still had residual bladder hyperactivity without infravesical obstruction. It can be assumed that 50% of detrusor hyperactivity in aging men generate primary hyperactivity irrespective of associated infravesical alterations, and 50% develop secondary hyperactivity due to infravesical obstruction. Deobstruction in these cases may causally treat aging men.

These results are supported by further urodynamic studies in Scandinavia investigating men with lower urinary tract symptoms before the operation. Although symptomatic, only 70% had a urodynamically proven infravesical obstruction and 37% showed detrusor hyperactivity. 30% did not have any sign of obstruction and required no surgery. These results emphasise the importance of thorough preoperative diagnostics in bladder outlet obstruction to optimise treatment outcome and therapeutic decisions.

It is well established that prostatic enlargement has two compartments:

1. the adenomyomatose hyperplasia of paraurethral glands, and
2. the fibromuscular compartment.

Both parts are under certain hormonal control; the glandular hyperplasia is regulated by androgens and the stromal part by oestrogens except the intraprostatic smooth muscle cells regulated by adrenergic stimuli. The use of antiandrogens results in notable epithelial cell apoptosis, a concept known since anti-androgen treatment for prostate cancer was established by Charles Huggins in the early 1950. More recent concepts on androgen metabolism in BPH suggested reduction in glandular compartment by blocking 5α-reductase, the key enzyme involved in intracellular dihydro-testosterone generation. Promising results of type 2 5α-reductase blockers (finasteride) in canine studies showed significant reduction of the glandular prostate volume. However, the canine prostate is predominantly characterised by glandular enlargement compared with the predominant stromal compartment in humans. Clinical studies in aging men reported prostate volume reduction, although long term data are currently not supporting the use of 5α-reductase blockers as widespread preventive drugs in aging men. This is related to the lack of correlation between prostate volume and grade of obstruction. A small median prostate lobe can cause more obstruction than a large adenoma extending to the rectum. In addition to these anatomical differences, prostate histology (myomatose or fibromatose) influences conservative outcome of outlet obstruction.

Phytopharmaca are assumed to improve detrusor hyperactivity via spasmolytic, antiphlogistic, and disinfectant effects. In addition to that, improvement of detrusor contractility has also been suggested. However, clinical studies have not proved these effects so far.

3.　　Summary

At present, treatment of the aging bladder should rely on antimuscarinics and behavioural training for detrusor hyperactivity, or, in the case of detrusor hypocontractility, cholinergics, α-blockers, catheterisation and surgical deobstruction after urodynamic studies. Before prescribing any medication for the aging bladder possible side effects and interactions with other medications must be considered. It should not be forgotten that reduction of medications often improves morbidity of elderly people.

We have recently reported on the positive effect of drug reduction in elderly patients, emphasising the importance of indication for treatment in this cohort. The combination of rising comorbidities and medications with their possible side effects should be evaluated carefully against the potential risks for aging men and women. Additionally the potential benefits and risks must be individually considered and evaluated with the patient to determine the best suitable treatment. A thorough history and investigation is mandatory in aging men and women before medications are prescribed. If that sequence is adhered to, even the common problems of the aging bladder will be treatable with success in most cases.

4.　　References

1. Abrams PH, Farrar DJ, Turner-Warwick RT, Whiteside CG, Feneley RC (1979) The results of prostatectomy: a symptomatic and urodynamic analysis of 152 patients. J Urol 121(5): 640–642
2. Chapple CR (2000) Muscarinic receptor antagonists in the treatment of overactive bladder. Urology 55[5A Suppl]: 33–46; discussion 50

3. Chapple CR, Yamanishi T, Chess-Williams R (2002) Muscarinic receptor subtypes and management of the overactive bladder. Urology 60[5 Suppl 1]: 82–88; discussion 88–89
4. Elbadawi A, Diokno AC, Millard RJ (1998) The aging bladder: morphology and urodynamics. World J Urol 16[Suppl 1]: S10–S34
5. Elbadawi A, Hailemariam S, Yalla SV, Resnick NM (1997a) Structural basis of geriatric voiding dysfunction. VI. Validation and update of diagnostic criteria in 71 detrusor biopsies. J Urol 157(5): 1802–1813
6. Elbadawi A, Hailemariam S, Yalla SV, Resnick NM (1997b) Structural basis of geriatric voiding dysfunction. VII. Prospective ultrastructural/urodynamic evaluation of its natural evolution. J Urol 157(5): 1814–1822
7. Elbadawi A, Yalla SV, Resnick NM (1993a) Structural basis of geriatric voiding dysfunction. I. Methods of a prospective ultrastructural/urodynamic study and an overview of the findings. J Urol 150(5 Pt 2): 1650–1656
8. Elbadawi A, Yalla SV, Resnick NM (1993b) Structural basis of geriatric voiding dysfunction. II. Aging detrusor: normal versus impaired contractility. J Urol 150(5 Pt 2): 1657–1667
9. Elbadawi A, Yalla SV, Resnick NM (1993c) Structural basis of geriatric voiding dysfunction. III. Detrusor overactivity. J Urol 150(5 Pt 2): 1668–1680
10. Elbadawi A, Yalla SV, Resnick NM (1993d) Structural basis of geriatric voiding dysfunction. IV. Bladder outlet obstruction. J Urol 150(5 Pt 2): 1681–1695
11. Gillberg PG, Sundquist S, Nilvebrant L (1998) Comparison of the in vitro and in vivo profiles of tolterodine with those of subtype-selective muscarinic receptor antagonists. Eur J Pharmacol 349(2–3): 285–292
12. Hailemariam S, Elbadawi A, Yalla SV, Resnick NM (1997) Structural basis of geriatric voiding dysfunction. V. Standardized protocols for routine ultrastructural study and diagnosis of endoscopic detrusor biopsies. J Urol 157(5): 1783–1801
13. Hegde SS, Eglen RM (1999) Muscarinic receptor subtypes modulating smooth muscle contractility in the urinary bladder. Life Sci 64(6–7): 419–428
14. Heslington K, Hilton P (1996) Ambulatory monitoring and conventional cystometry in asymptomatic female volunteers. Br J Obstet Gynaecol 103(5): 434–441
15. Ikeda K, Kobayashi S, Suzuki M et al (2002) M(3) receptor antagonism by the novel antimuscarinic agent solifenacin in the urinary bladder and salivary gland. Naunyn Schmiedebergs Arch Pharmacol 366(2): 97–103
16. Kiwamoto H, Ma FH, Higashira H, Park YC, Kurita T (2001) Identification of muscarinic receptor subtypes of cultured smooth muscle cells and tissue of human bladder body. Int J Urol 8(10): 557–563
17. Palmer J (1983) Report of a double-blind crossover study of flurbiprofen and placebo in detrusor instability. J Int Med Res 11[Suppl 2]: 11–17
18. Thüroff JW, Chartier-Kastler E, Corcus J, Humke J, Jonas U, Palmtag H, Tanagho EA (1998) Medical treatment and medical side effects in urinary incontinence in the elderly. World J Urol 16[Suppl 1]: S48–S61

Correspondence address: Christian Hampel, MD, Department of Urology, Johannes Gutenberg University Mainz, Langenbeckstrasse 1, D-55131 Mainz (E-mail: hampel@urologie.klinik.uni-mainz.de).

Hormonal replacement therapy for the aging bladder

E. Plas and *L. K. Daha*

Department of Urology and LBI for Urology & Andrology,
Lainz Hospital Vienna, Vienna

Contents

1.   Introduction

Aging is accompanied by the development of various, sometimes distressing, symptoms of different organ systems including the genitourinary tract. Alterations of the genitourinary tract are common during aging, with sex specific differences, that is, the development of irritative bladder symptoms both in men and women, stress incontinence more often reported by women, and bladder outlet obstruction in aging men.

The prevalence of bladder symptoms for aging men and women is known to be high, but, although commonly reported, only 60% of patients looked for relief and treatment (Milsom et al. 2001). Complaints from urinary frequency, urgency, dysuria, nocturia, genuine stress- and/or urge incontinence are regularly stated. However, the most often reported symptoms are urgency and urge incontinence. Questionnaires sent to more than 3000 European women aged 55–75 years showed that 30% suffered from genitourinary symptoms, most commonly frequency (12.7%), vaginal itching (10.6%), dysuria (8.3%), incontinence (7.4%), and recurrent urinary tract infections in 7.4% (Barlow et al. 1997). Overall, 60% of these women made efforts to alleviate their symptoms and looked for help.

The reason for the development of bladder symptoms are multifactorial and result from morphological and functional alterations of the bladder.

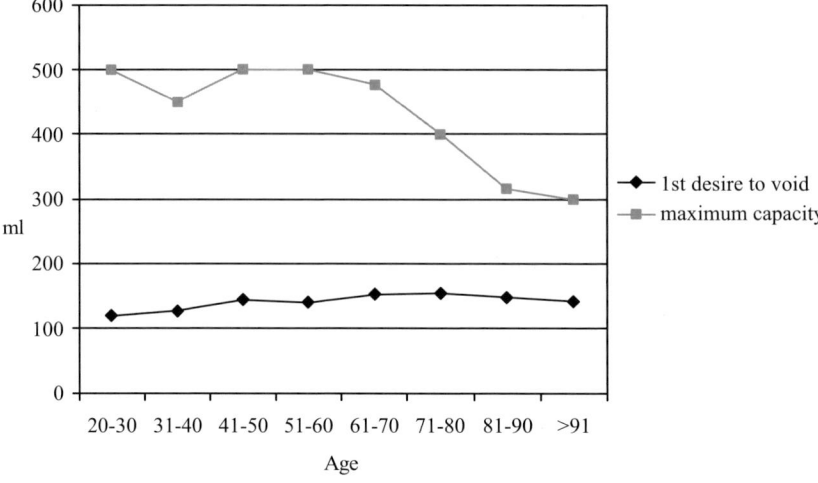

Fig. 1. Urodynamic investigations in women between 20–90 years by Collas and Malone-Lee (Collas and Malone-Lee 1996). As shown, there is a constant increase in 1st desire to void associated with a decrease in maximum bladder capacity with aging

Besides the development of morphological alterations of the aging detrusor, Collas and Malone-Lee found functional changes of the bladder detrusor with aging (Collas and Malone-Lee 1996). Urodynamic investigations in more than 1300 women aged 20–90 years showed a significant reduction in bladder compliance and maximal capacity associated with an increase in bladder capacity at first desire to void (Fig. 1) (Collas and Malone-Lee 1996).

These alterations during the filling phase are related to urgency and sometimes urge incontinence. The high incidence of urgency in aging men and women causes embarrassment due to fear of incontinence. This, in turn, is often associated with reduction in social activities – for example, shopping is planned according to the availability of toilets, cultural events are avoided because of lack of toilets, etc. Restriction of private activities can result in hermit-like isolation and depression requiring antidepressive medication in many cases.

In addition to changes in the aging detrusor, comorbidity of neurological, endocrine, and orthopaedic disorders, diabetes, and heart disease are increasing with aging. The increase in comorbidity requires medical treatment, which in many cases affects detrusor function. Further, chronic constipation in aging men and women and its treatment may also influence function of the lower genitourinary tract.

Increasing costs of healthcare systems worldwide are of major concern; it is well known that 90% of individual health expenses are spent in people's last 10 years of life. With the proposed development of world population and the increasing percentage of people older than 60 years, economy is faced with unresolved questions concerning health costs and budgets.

A tremendous amount of expenses are used for antidepressive medications and incontinence devices.

Keeping this in mind, it is extremely important to look for further strategies for the treatment and/or prevention of the aging detrusor. This will be not only of notable impact for the patient but also for healthcare budgets.

2.   Hormonal aspects and aging

Aging is accompanied by alterations of testicular and ovarian function leading to hormonal changes both in men and in women.

2.1   Hormones and men

In aging men, continuous reduction in total testosterone, free testosterone, DHEA, DHEAS and growth hormone have been reported by Gray et al. with an onset from age 45 years (Gray et al. 1991). However, hypogonadism defined by serum total testosterone <3 ng/ml will be found in only 7% of men aged 45–60, 25% at 60–80 years, and 33% in men older than 80 years (Vermeulen and Kaufman 1995). Although Neaves et al. reported a decrease in Leydig cells correlating with age, no clear correlation of decreasing Leydig cells and testosterone has been shown (Neaves et al. 1984). Additionally, a decrease in Leydig cells and testosterone may suggest a reduction of spermatogenesis in aging men. But recent reports showed a life-long persistence of spermatogenesis and fertility in healthy aging men irrespective of age (Plas et al. 2000, Rolf and Nieschlag 2001).

Although hormonal changes in aging men are well established, investigations concerning possible correlations of androgens and detrusor function are barely available. In a recent report, the effect of androgens on urodynamics in intersex female patients was studied (Celayir et al. 2000). A reduced bladder capacity of androgenised female patients was found in relation to age, suggesting an antagonistic effect of androgens on bladder urodynamics in intersex females with adrenogenital syndromes (Celayir et al. 2000). A direct effect of testosterone and castration in the male urinary rabbit detrusor on autonomic receptor density and contractility was investigated by Anderson and Navarro (Anderson and Navarro 1988). An alteration in muscarinic cholinergic receptor density was found, with no change in α-adrenergic or β-adrenergic receptor density. It was concluded that castration downregulates α-adrenergic receptors of the bladder base, whereas testosterone treatment increases the density of muscarinic cholinergic receptors and increases the ratio of bladder to total body weight. Although no contractile changes were observed in the bladder base tissue in relation to testosterone concentration, it was suggested that longer chronic testosterone deficits might affect bladder outlet resistance in men because of the reduced α-adrenergic receptor density (Anderson and Navarro 1988).

In addition to these results, Keast and Saunders reported on morphological effects of autonomic nerves supplying visceral organs in pre- and postpubertally castrated male rats (Keast and Saunders 1998). After castration, noradrenergic pelvic neurons supplying the vas deferens, prostate, urinary bladder, and colon achieved only 60% of the size compared with controls. Cholinergic pelvic neurons were unaffected by castration. The interesting finding was that testosterone replacement in castrated rats prevented these changes. It was suggested that androgens are essential for maturation and maintenance of groups of autonomic neurons supplying pelvic organs (Keast and Saunders 1998). Whether these data are of clinical relevance can only be speculated but it may open new areas of clinical research concerning neural supply of pelvic organs in testosterone deficient male patients.

2.2   Hormones and women

The withdrawal of ovarian function by entering menopause is well defined and can be easily proved by blood sampling (Table 1) (Cobin et al. 1999). However, urogenital symptoms are usually not abundant at entering menopause but may occur few years later and persist throughout lifetime (Samsioe 1998). Since female aging is associated with reduction in serum estradiol and its metabolites and aging is related with increasing symptoms of urgency, vaginal burning and itching, incontinence, dysuria, nocturia, and recurrent urinary tract infections, a correlation of hormonal reduction with the development of lower genitourinary tract symptoms appears plausible.

Although an association of oestrogen deficiency and symptoms of the lower urinary tract is likely, only few randomised, controlled data are available.

Table 1. Hormonal investigations for determination of menopause, modified after American Association of Clinical Endocrinology Guidelines 1999

FSH	>40 IU/l
LH	>10 IU/l
Estradiol	<30 pg/ml

3.   Hormones and the genitourinary tract

Since there are no clinical studies on hormone replacement therapy (HRT) and bladder function available in aging men, this review will only focus on effects of hormone replacement on the lower genitourinary tract in aging women. The main hormones in the female genitourinary tract are oestrogen and progesterone. Embryological, the bladder, urethra, and distal portion of the vagina differentiate from the urogenital sinus and develop out of the cloacae.

3.1   Oestrogen

Oestrogen receptors are found in the lower genitourinary tract except in the transitional epithelium of the bladder, apart from trigonal areas that underwent squamous metaplasia (Hextall 2000). The concentration of oestrogen receptors in the bladder is considerably lower than in the urethra and vagina. It is therefore not surprising to find similar hormonal receptors and effects both in the urethra and vagina but not in the bladder. Besides the presence of oestrogen receptors in the urethra and vagina, they have also been identified in the pubococcygeus muscle of the pelvic floor (Hextall 2000, Elia and Bergman 1993).

Because of the number of different sites of action, oestrogens have been shown to increase urethral closure pressure and improve pressure transmission to the urethra in the non-obese women. Further, an increased blood flow in the uterus, vagina, and urethra has been found after intraarterial injection of estradiol (Batra et al. 1985, Batra et al. 1986) and dilation of blood vessels surrounding the urethra (Yokoyama et al. 1983). In addition to these perfusive effects of organs developing from the urogenital sinus, oestrogen has also been associated with an increase in proliferation of superficial squamous epithelial cells (Bergman et al. 1990, Ulmsten and Stormby 1987), which supports a trophic epithelial action (Kuroda et al. 1985). These oestrogenic effects can be observed regularly in cycling women (women who have regular menstrual bleeding), combined with cyclical changes of urinary and vaginal cytology. Besides these effects, oestrogens may directly influence smooth muscle cell activity and responsiveness to adrenergic receptors. An oestrogen induced increased sensitivity of adrenergic receptors has been attributed to an increase in number of postjunctional α_2-adrenoreceptors, causing contraction of the periurethral smooth muscle (Larsson et al. 1984). Additionally, a direct effect of oestrogen on the rat detrusor, with reduction in amplitude and frequency of spontaneous rhythmic contractions, has been reported (Shenfield et al. 1998). However, oestrogens may not only have a direct effect on the detrusor but an age dependent response to exogenous oestrogen on micturition, contractility, and cholinergic receptors was also suggested (Diep and Constantinou 1999). Diep and Constantinou studied the effect of ovarectomy and 17ß-estradiol supplementation on urodynamics and responsiveness to cholinergic stimulation at different ages (Diep and Constantinou 1999). They found different responses between detrusors in young and mature rats to exogenous oestrogen, which implies that endogenous oestrogen may be of major importance in the neuromuscular development of normal bladder function and micturition reflexes (Diep and Constantinou 1999).

Investigations on detrusor contractility showed that ovarectomy in young rats irreversibly decreased the response to cholinergic stimulation. It was hypothesized that exogenous oestrogen may partially restore function of the young rat detrusor whereas in mature rats, exogenous oestrogen was able to reverse the effects of ovarectomy (Diep and Constantinou 1999). These findings suggested an impact of oestrogen on bladder function depending on the age at which it was applied.

The clinical relevance of these findings were summarised by Samsioe and Nillson as presented in Figs. 2 and 3 (Samsioe 1998, Nilsson 1994). Because of the progressive decline in oestrogen during the menopause,

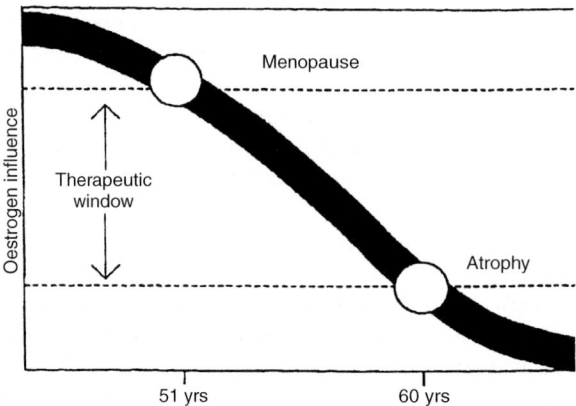

Fig. 2. Progressive decline of estrogens during climacteric contribute to atrophy-related urogenital symptoms. These symptoms typically occur later than vasomotor symptoms and often considerably later than menopause itself. It is possible to administer estrogens to combat urogenital estrogen deficiency symptoms without inducing endometrial growth (reprinted with permission [Samsioe 1998])

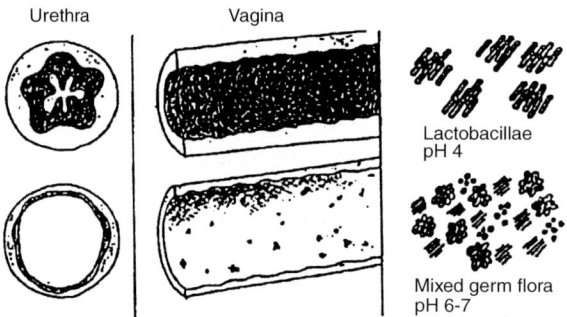

Fig. 3. Climacteric alterations of the urethra and vagina during menopause as a result of estrogen deficiency. As shown, there are not only changes in epithelial thickness but also in vaginal pH and flora with decrease in lactobacilli and increase in uropathogens (Nilsson 1994)

atrophy of urethral and vaginal epithelium occurs concomitant with reductions in submucosal and periurethral connective tissue. This, in turn, results in a diminished support of the urethra and its continence mechanism.

Female continence is maintained by interaction of several anatomic structures, including the striated sphincter, urethral circular and longitudinal smooth muscle, submucosal vasculature, urethral epithelium and, extraurethrally, the pelvic floor (Hextall 2000, Elia and Bergman 1993, Andersson et al. 1999). In addition to that, the menopause results in alterations of vaginal epithelium, reductions in the thickening of vaginal mucosa, and decreases in lactobacilli (Nilsson 1994). These changes lead to an increased vaginal pH and development of pathogenic organisms, which can cause vaginal symptoms and recurrent urinary tract infections (Barlow et al. 1997, Hextall 2000, Fantl 1994, Kok et al. 1999, Raz and Stamm 1993).

The importance of oestrogens for the genitourinary tract is well established and support a possible role of hormone replacement in the prevention of bladder and vaginal symptoms during aging.

3.2   Progesterone

In addition to the evidence of oestrogen action on the urethra, vagina and parts of the bladder, progesterone receptors were also determined in the urethra, vagina, bladder and pelvic floor (Hextall 2000, Rizk et al. 2001). Some evidence suggest an involvement of progesterone in the development of urinary symptoms.

Urodynamic investigations in pregnant women determined increased bladder capacity and compliance correlating positively with increased serum progesterone (Rizk et al. 2001, Cardozo and Kelleher 1995). In cycling women, urgency and frequency were reported to become worse just before menstrual bleeding (Shimonovitz et al. 1997). Additionally, detrusor instability has been shown to correlate with time from the last menstrual bleeding in cycling women (Hextall et al. 2001). These clinical findings are consistent with an increased frequency but reduced amplitude of contractions of detrusor smooth muscle strips after administration of progesterone in vitro (Shenfeld et al. 1999).

Progesterone is considered an antagonist to estrogen mediating its effect by reduction of oestrogen receptors in target organs (Rizk et al. 2001). It has been hypothesized that deficiency of progesterone could affect urethral resistance and/or bladder compliance in women similarly to estrogen (Rizk et al. 2001). However, the action of progesterone in the aging female genitourinary tract is not completely understood yet, although it has been suggested that progesterone action may predominate at receptor levels in the bladder resulting in suppression of estrogen receptors (Batra and Iosif 1987).

4.   Hormonal replacement therapy in the aging female

Due to the presence of oestrogen and progesterone receptors in the lower genitourinary tract and pelvic floor and the proven deficiency of these hormones during menopause, hormone replacement seems plausible for the treatment of the symptomatic postmenopausal women. The first trial on hormone replacement in postmenopausal women was reported by Salmon et al. in 1944, investigating the effect of oestrogen for the treatment of dysuria and incontinence (Salmon et al. 1941). Although this was more than 50 years ago, the question still remains whether there is objective improvement of postmenopausal women with genitourinary complaints in prospective controlled trials.

The presence of personal experiences often prohibits scientific investigations of obviously clear outcomes. Because of this and its expected outcome analysis, randomised controlled trials for critical assessing the role of hormone replacement unto urgency, incontinence, vaginal itching, and burning sensations, dyspareunia, etc, have been performed only rarely. Numerous uncontrolled, case record trials have been performed and analysed retrospectively, supporting a beneficial effect of oestrogens for the aging bladder. But only few randomised, controlled trials were performed, and these reported contradictory results.

In a meta-analysis of the Hormones and Urogenital Therapy Committee published in 1996, it was clearly shown that most of the data concerning hormone replacement in aging women came from non-randomised, uncontrolled trials (Fantl et al. 1994). Out of 166 articles on oestrogen replacement monotherapy or combined replacement of oestrogen/progesterone in women with stress-, urge- or mixed incontinence, only six were controlled, randomised trials (3.6%) and 17/166 were uncontrolled clinical series (10.2%) (Fantl et al. 1994). Most publications (86.2%) were uncontrolled retrospective series. This imbalance in high quality papers and papers of less scientific relevance undermines the importance of controlled, randomised, prospective trials for clarifying clinical questions even more than 50 years after the first trial on hormone replacement in symptomatic women.

Although six prospective controlled, randomised trials with urodynamic investigations have been performed (Henalla et al. 1988, Judge 1969, Samsioe et al. 1985, Wilson et al. 1987, Walter et al. 1978, Walter et al. 1990), another important issue in the evaluation of efficacy of hormone replacement in postmenopausal women was shown by the Hormones and Urogenital Therapy Committee, namely, heterogeneity of inclusion criteria and patients investigated (Fantl et al. 1994). Overall 159 patients were included in these trials, 92 patients (58%) had genuine stress incontinence, 59 cases (37%) had urgency and 8 women (5%) had mixed incontinence. Besides the large variety of urodynamic findings and indications for treatment, variations were also present in treatment duration (1–4 months), medications (conjugated equine oestrogen, esterified oestrogen, estropipate, 17ß-estradiol, ethinyl estradiol), route of application (oral or vaginal), and dosages. The heterogeneity in study populations makes clear conclusions on the use of hormone replacement in these cases difficult.

Analysing clinical outcome, subjective improvement under hormone replacement was observed in 64–75% compared with placebo, with improvement rates of 10–56%. The difference between the verum and placebo groups ranged from 19–89%, suggesting a positive effect of hormone replacement. Five of the six controlled studies reported significant improvement of symptoms, with no objective improvement determined by urodynamics.

In uncontrolled series, overall 523 women were investigated with genuine stress incontinence in 36.2%, detrusor instability in 11.1%, and mixed incontinence in 52.6% (Fantl et al. 1994). Again treatment regimes, duration of therapy (1–120 months), and applications were different in most studies. Oestrogen treatment improved symptoms in 8–89%, with an overall estimated benefit for all forms of bladder symptoms in 64%. If patients who only had stress incontinence were considered, the estimated improvement rate was 53%.

Patients experienced relief or improvement of symptoms quite often, but data on the quantity of fluid loss were scarce. Only Henalla et al. reported significant improvement in loss of fluid after HRT whereas data from others reached minor significance or non-significant findings (Henalla et al. 1988).

In conclusion, the Hormones and Urogenital Therapy Committee stated that there is no strong evidence for a beneficial effect of oestrogen treatment concerning objective outcome and change in urodynamics in aging women, although subjective improvement was seen regularly in women taking oestrogens and placebo (Fantl et al. 1994).

Further randomised, double blind, placebo controlled results were added by Fantl et al. in 83 hypoestrogenic women with genuine stress- or urge incontinence and mixed symptoms (Fantl et al. 1996). Mean duration of menopause was 11 years, with a mean estradiol (E2) concentration at baseline of 9 pg/ml. Women in the verum group received 0.625 mg oestrogen and 10 mg medroxyprogesterone cyclically for three months. Patients underwent urodynamics before and after treatment. Although normal E2 levels for cycling women were achieved (mean 61 pg/ml), only 54% of women receiving HRT reported an improvement of incontinence compared with 45% in the placebo group (P > 0.05). Objective outcome measurement on incontinence episodes, fluid loss, and the number of diurnal and nocturnal voluntary micturitions were not significantly different. Additionally, questionnaires concerning quality of life did not show any difference between the groups (Fantl et al. 1996). In a recent placebo controlled trial, 63 postmenopausal women with genuine stress incontinence received oestrogen supplementation (2 mg oestradiol-valerate daily) for six months. This showed no beneficial outcome compared with placebo (Jackson et al. 1999). Duration of menopause in these women ranged between mean 12.2–13.5 years. Consistent with urodynamic findings from Collas and Malone-Lee, volume at first desire to void was increased (179–219 ml) and bladder capacity reduced in these women (Collas and Malone-Lee 1996). The issue of patients' compliance was specifically addressed and reported as high (> 80%). However, no subjective and/or objective improvement was observed. Besides, the negative outcome of hormone replacement on detrusor function, a positive effect on sexual function with decrease in dyspareunia, pain due to vaginal dryness, and reduction in incontinence during intercourse was reported (Jackson et al. 1999). Consistent with previous reports, no significant benefit of hormone replacement for genuine stress incontinence in the postmenopausal women was found.

As already mentioned, the need of incontinence devices and costs rises significantly with aging, especially for elderly people living in nursing homes. This issue was specifically addressed by Ouslander et al., who looked at the effect of hormone replacement in female nursing home residents (Ouslander et al. 2001). In a randomised, placebo controlled trial, 32 incontinent women (average age 88 years) received hormone replacement (0.625 mg oestrogen oral and progesterone 2.5 mg) or placebo daily for six months. On the basis of clinical assessment only, all subjects complained predominately of urge incontinence, except for three women with mixed incontinence. After 6 months of systemic treatment, wetness rates, fluid loss, and bladder capacity in the groups were not different. Urethral and vaginal smears showed a beneficial but no significant effect of HRT on urethra and vaginal atrophy with an increase in the proportion of superficial cells (Ouslander et al. 2001). During treatment, vaginal pH declined from 5.9 to 5.5, suggesting a positive effect of local oestrogen treatment. However, complete restoration of vaginal and/or urethral epithelium was not achieved by hormone replacement. Even in this highly selected cohort of elderly women in nursing homes, hormonal replacement was of no benefit for incontinence treatment but potentially beneficial in improving local symptoms (vaginal dryness, itching, recurrent infections) (Ouslander et al. 2001).

The largest prospective trial on the efficacy of postmenopausal hormonal replacement for the prevention or improvement of genitourinary symptoms result from a subanalysis of the Heart and Estrogen/Progestin Replacement study (Grady et al. 2001). In this study, 2763 postmenopausal women with coronary heart disease were investigated. 55% (n = 1520) reported at least one episode of incontinence per week. These women were randomly assigned to daily oestrogen (0.625 mg) and medroxyprogesterone acetate (2.5 mg) or placebo and followed for a mean of 4.1 years. Symptoms and incontinence were classified by questionnaires only, urodynamic studies were not performed. At baseline, urge incontinence was reported by 26%, genuine stress incontinence by 23%, and mixed incontinence by 51%. During treatment, 26% in the placebo group improved compared with 20.9% in the hormone replacement group, whereas 27% of women receiving placebo deteriorated compared with 38.8% under estrogen/progesterone substitution (Fig. 4). Again, no significant benefit of hormone replacement on incontinence in postmenopausal women was found, which leads to the conclusion that there is no rationale for oestrogen replacement in postmenopausal women for the treatment of incontinence (Grady et al. 2001).

Only, Kok et al. recently reported a beneficial effect of hormone replacement (2 mg 17β-estradiol with 2.5 mg, 5 mg, 10 mg, or 15 mg dydrogesterone daily) in 95 postmenopausal women (Kok et al. 1999). In an uncontrolled series, 23.3% were cured after 6 months of hormone replacement, and 65.4% experienced disappearance of nocturia. The different doses of progesterone did not of effect daytime and night time voiding.

Another aspect influencing the outcome of hormone replacement can be the variable endogenous oestrogen status of elderly women. Highly variable levels of oestrogens are present in nearly all postmenopausal women, even

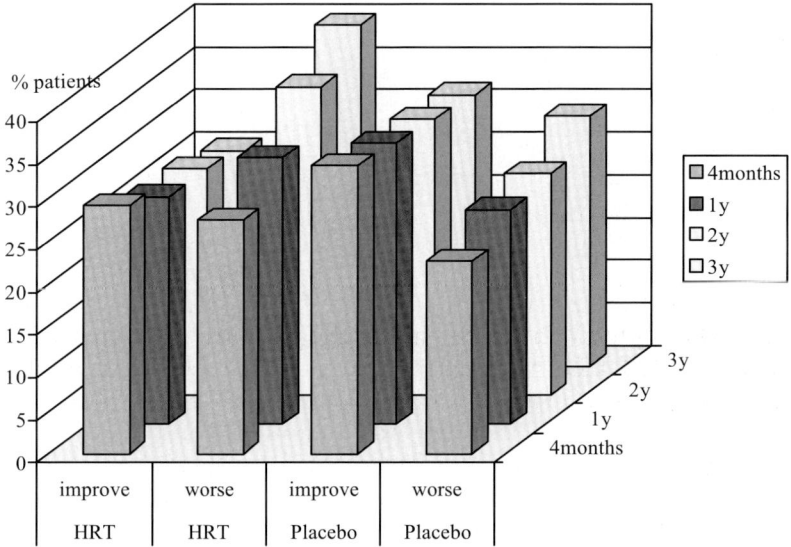

Fig. 4. Changes (%) in severity of urinary incontinence during 3 year follow-up reported by Grady et al. (2001). As shown, there was a significant increase in the estrogen treated group as compared to placebo

at advanced ages (Kuchel et al. 2001). Similar to other endocrine systems, oestrogen deficiency and the need for its replacement are, therefore, likely to be relative rather than absolute. Because many markers of oestrogen deficiency overlap between risk groups, their clinical usefulness for deciding whether hormone replacement will be beneficial or not is limited. It will be important to look for additional markers of overall estrogenic effects at the target tissues, for example karyopyknotic index on vaginal wall smear, vaginal pH testing (Kuchel et al. 2001, Notelovitz 1995).

5.   Complications of hormonal replacement therapy

Although hormone replacement is a well tolerated treatment, patients must be well informed and aware of possible side effects. Oestrogen substitution can be associated with breakthrough bleeding, which has been reported in up to 20% of postmenopausal women (Jackson et al. 1999). This may be avoided with the addition of continuous or intermittent application of progesterone. Women who have not had a hysterectomy and are taking oestrogen replacement require some form of progesterone opposition in any case.

In addition to breakthrough bleeding, oestrogen therapy may be associated with an increased risk of cancer of the breast and endometrium. The incidence of breast cancer under systemic oestrogen replacement was shown to be considerable and not reduced by the addition of proges- terone (Colditz et al. 1995). Colditz et al. found an increased risk for cancer development among postmenopausal women taking oestrogen

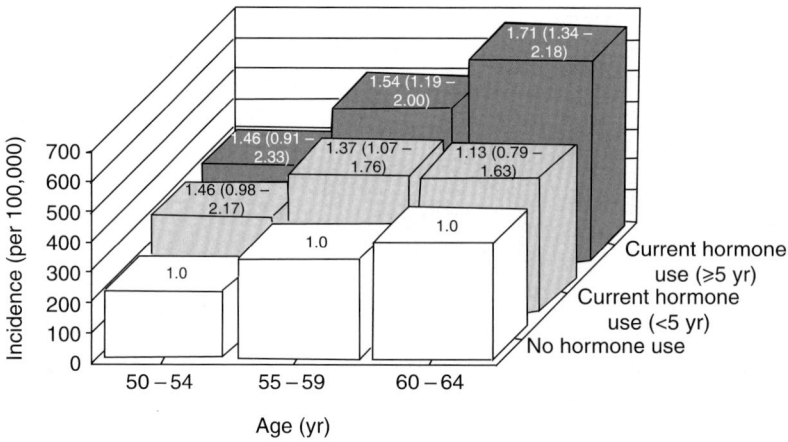

Fig. 5. Incidence and relative risk of breast cancer according to age and the duration of current postmenopausal hormone therapy (reprinted with permission [Colditz et al. 1995]; Copyright ownership 1995, Massachusetts Medical Society, all rights reserved)

monotherapy and combination therapy compared with women who had never taken any hormonal treatment (Colditz et al. 1995). Incidence in breast cancer correlated positively with duration of therapy, in women taking oestrogen therapy for less than five years the risk of developing cancer was lower compared with hormone replacement for more than 5–10 years. Additionally, older women taken hormone replacement for more than five years were at greater risk for cancer development (Fig. 5) (Colditz et al. 1995). Among current users of hormone replacement or those who stopped 1–4 years ago, the relative risk of developing breast cancer increased by 1.023 for each year of hormone use (Genazzani et al. 2001). Recent data suggested that an oestrogen-progestin regimen may increase the risk of breast cancer beyond that associated with oestrogen alone. However, the effect of progestogens on the breast remains unclear so far. Due to the slightly increased risk of breast cancer development, oestrogen replacement is contraindicated in women with breast cancer that is positive for oestrogen receptors (Genazzani et al. 2001).

The risk of cancer development may be reduced by transvaginal application of estrogens. Pharmacokinetic studies on transvaginal oestrogen applied as creams or pessaries showed minor systemic absorption of oestrogen compared with systemic application (Samsioe 1998, Nilsson and Heimer 1992, Bachmann 1995). However, long term data regarding cancer risk in these cases are missing. Since vaginal dryness, itching, and urgency are related with atrophy of the external genitalia in aging women, local treatment can be recommended except in women with receptor positive breast cancer.

Besides breast cancer, endometrium cancer also may be related to hormone replacement. Grady et al. investigated the association of unopposed oestrogen or oestrogen plus progestin treatment and the risk of developing endometrial cancer (Grady et al. 1995). In a meta-analysis, the risk was found to increase significantly with duration of unopposed oestrogen treatment. This risk persisted for several years after discontinuation of oestrogen replacement (Grady et al. 1995). Unopposed oestrogen replacement is known to increase the risk of developing endometrial cancer and is therefore appropriate only for women who have had hysterectomies.

To decrease the risk of endometrial hyperstimulation, an adequate dose of progestin should be given in a continuous combined regimen or for an appropriate number of days (10–12 days). Among women receiving combination treatment (oestrogen plus progestin), cohort studies showed a decreased risk in endometrial cancer whereas case-control studies reported a slight increase, which shows the conflicting data that are available. Hormone replacement is generally considered to be contraindicated in patients with endometrial cancer.

In order to minimise the risk of endometrial cancer, Jackson et al. suggested transvaginal ultrasound before treatment to determine the thickness of the endometrium (Jackson et al. 1999). If the endometrium is less than 4 mm women were considered as candidates for hormone replacement.

Since the beneficial effects of hormone replacement in postmenopausal women are still controversial, its possible benefits and risks have to be carefully assessed and discussed with the patient before starting either mono- or combined oestrogen replacement therapy.

6. Hormonal replacement therapy and urinary tract infections in women

Urinary tract infections are common in women, particularly in elderly women, with an incidence of 20–50% compared with 1% in adolescents (Sandford 1975, Boscia and Kaye 1987). The reasons for the increased frequency in postmenopausal women are multifactorial and include impairment of bladder emptying, incontinence, constipation, poor hygiene, changes of vaginal flora and pH. Postmenopausal oestrogen deficiency leads to atrophy of the vaginal mucosa, with reduction of lactobacilli and immediate establishment of gram-negative bacteria (Hextall 2000). Additional to that, microlesions of the vagina mucosal due to dryness can cause petechial bleeding during intercourse (Samsioe 1998). This may lead to partial vaginal obliteration most pronounced in the fundal region of the vagina. As a result, itching and burning sensations are common, often associated with an odour from contamination of the vagina with pathogenic bacteria.

Local application of oestrogen may be beneficial to prevent mucosal atrophy and improve vaginal symptoms. In a randomised study in 108 postmenopausal women with recurrent urinary tract infections, women were randomly assigned to transvaginal 7.5 mcg estradiol for 24 hours or no treatment (Eriksen 1999). After 36 weeks of treatment, the cumulative probability to remain free of infection was 45% in women taking hormone replacement compared with 20% of women receiving no treatment (Eriksen 1999). Raz et al. investigated the use of intravaginal estriol (0.5 mg) cream in 93 postmenopausal women, again finding a significant reduction in urinary tract infections compared with placebo (Raz and Stamm 1993). Lactobacilli were absent in all cultures before treatment and reappeared after one month of treatment in 61% in the oestrogen group but not in the controls. Additionally, vaginal pH declined after one month of treatment from baseline 5.5 to 3.8 during hormone replacement. After four months of treatment, the cumulative likelihood to remain free of disease was 0.95 in the oestrogen group compared with 0.3 in controls. Overall, patients taking hormone replacement required significantly fewer antibiotics during the study period compared with controls (Raz and Stamm 1993).

In a recent systemic meta-analysis the effect of oestrogen supplementation in the prevention of recurrent urinary tract infections in postmenopausal women was investigated (Cardozo et al. 2001). Meta-analysis from 334 women showed a significant benefit from oestrogen replacement over placebo, especially in those trials that studied local hormone supplementation. It was concluded that vaginal administration of oestrogens seems to be effective in the prevention of recurrent urinary tract infections in postmenopausal women (Cardozo et al. 2001).

7. Closing remarks

Alterations of bladder function occur during aging as a result of morphological and functional changes both in men and in women. These changes can be distressing and of significant negative impact on quality of life because of urgency, frequency, nocturia, and incontinence. Concomitant with alterations of bladder function hormonal changes occur in women with the termination of ovarian function and continuous decline in androgen production in men. Therefore, a regulatory influence of hormones unto the genitourinary tract is plausible. The data on androgen interaction with detrusor function are scarce, and no clinical report is available on direct action of androgens on the aging male detrusor so far. Contrary to that, numerous trials have addressed the issue of hormone replacement in postmenopausal women. Analysing only uncontrolled trials and personal experiences suggest a beneficial effect of oestrogen replacement for incontinence. However, only a few, randomised controlled studies on oestrogen replacement were reported in aging women, which showed no significant effect of hormone replacement in the relief of genuine stress- and urge incontinence. Therefore hormonal replacement cannot be recommended for the treatment of incontinence in postmenopausal women. Vaginal itching and dryness causing dyspareunia can be treated successfully with local oestrogen application, without any side effects and low risk of breast and endometrium cancer. Hormone replacement in postmenopausal women may also be beneficial for recurrent urinary tract infections by lowering vaginal pH, decontamination with gram-negative bacteria, and increasing number of lactobacilli.

It will be interesting to know if the duration of menopause may influence the value of hormone replacement in aging women and if early substitution may be able to prevent local symptoms of oestrogen deficiency. This issue should be addressed in future studies. Although numerous studies on hormone replacement have been already performed in the past 60 years randomised, controlled trials are needed to determine the role of oestrogen replacement for the detrusor in aging women. Endocrinology in aging men and women will become of considerable importance in future work on therapeutic aspects and new strategies to enable healthy aging, with a high quality of life for the aging person.

8.   References

1. Anderson GF, Navarro SP (1988) The response of autonomic receptors to castration and testosterone in the urinary bladder of the rabbit. J Urol 140: 885–889
2. Andersson KE, Appell R, Cardozo LD, Chapple C, Drutz HP, Finkbeiner AE, Haab F, Vela Navarrete R (1999) The pharmacological treatment of urinary incontinence. BJU Int 84: 923–947
3. Bachmann G (1995) The estradiol vaginal ring – a study of existing clinical data. Maturitas 22: S21–S29
4. Barlow DH, Samsioe G, van Geelen JM (1997) A study of European womens' experience of the problems of urogenital aging and its management. Maturitas 27: 239–247
5. Batra S, Bjellin L, Iosif S, Martensson L, Sjogren C (1985) Effect of oestrogen and progesterone on the blood flow in the lower urinary tract of the rabbit. Acta Physiol Scand 123: 191–194
6. Batra S, Bjellin L, Sjogren C, Iosif S, Widmark E (1986) Increases in blood flow of the female rabbit urethra following low dose estrogens. J Urol 136: 1360–1362
7. Batra SC, Iosif CS (1987) Progesterone receptors in the female lower urinary tract. J Urol 138: 1301–1304
8. Bergman A, Karram MM, Bhatia NN (1990) Changes in urethral cytology following estrogen administration. Gynecol Obstet Invest 29(3): 211–213
9. Boscia JA, Kaye D (1987) Asymptomatic bacteriuria in the elderly. Infect Dis Clin North Am 1: 893–905
10. Cardozo LD, Kelleher CJ (1995) Sex hormones, the menopause and urinary problems. Gynecol Endocrinol 9: 75–84
11. Cardozo L, Lose G, McClish D, Versi E, de Koning Gans H (2001) A systematic review of estrogens for recurrent urinary tract infections: third report of the hormones and urogenital therapy (HUT) committee. Int Urogynecol J Pelvic Floor Dysfunct 12: 15–20
12. Celayir S, Ilce Z, Danismend N (2000) Effects of male sex hormones on urodynamics in childhood: intersex patients are a natural model. Pediatr Surg Int 16: 502–504

13. Cobin RH, Bedsoe MB, Futerweit W, Goldzieher JW, Goodman NF, Petak SM, Smith KD, Steinberger E (1999) AACE Medical Guidelines for clinical practice for management of menopause. Endocrine Practice 5: 354–366

14. Colditz GA, Hankinson SE, Hunter DJ, Willett WC, Manson JE, Stampfer MJ, Hennekens C, Rosner B, Speizer FE (1995) The use of estrogens and progestins and the risk of breast cancer in postmenopausal women. N Engl J Med 332: 1589–1593

15. Collas DM, Malone-Lee JG (1996) Age-associated changes in detrusor sensory function in women with lower urinary tract symptoms. Int Urogynecol J Pelvic Floor Dysfunct 7: 24–29

16. Diep N, Constantinou CE (1999) Age dependent response to exogenous estrogen on micturition, contractility and cholinergic receptors of the rat bladder. Life Sci 64: PL 279–289

17. Elia G, Bergman A (1993) Estrogen effects on the urethra: beneficial effects in women with genuine stress incontinence. Obstet Gynecol Surv 48: 509–517

18. Eriksen B (1999) A randomized, open, parallel-group study on the preventive effect of an estradiol-releasing vaginal ring (Estring) on recurrent urinary tract infections in postmenopausal women. Am J Obstet Gynecol 180: 1072–1079

19. Fantl JA (1994) The lower urinary tract in women – effect of aging and menopause on continence. Exp Gerontol 29: 417–422

20. Fantl JA, Bump RC, Robinson D, McClish DK, Wyman JF (1996) Efficacy of estrogen supplementation in the treatment of urinary incontinence. The Continence Program for Women Research Group. Obstet Gynecol 88: 745–749

21. Fantl JA, Cardozo L, McClish DK (1994) Estrogen therapy in the management of urinary incontinence in postmenopausal women: a meta-analysis. First report of the Hormones and Urogenital Therapy Committee. Obstet Gynecol 83: 12–18

22. Genazzani AR, Gadducci A, Gambacciani M (2001) Controversial issues in climacteric medicine II. Hormone replacement therapy and cancer. International Menopause Society Expert Workshop. Climacteric 4: 181–193

23. Grady D, Brown JS, Vittinghoff E, Applegate W, Varner E, Snyder T, The HERS Research Group (2001) Postmenopausal hormones and incontinence: the Heart and Estrogen/Progestin Replacement Study. Obstet Gynecol 97: 116–120

24. Grady D, Gebretsadik T, Kerlikowske K, Ernster V, Petitti D (1995) Hormone replacement therapy and endometrial cancer risk: a meta-analysis. Obstet Gynecol 85: 304–313

25. Gray A, Feldman HA, McKinlay JB, Longcope C (1991) Age, disease, and changing sex hormone levels in middle-aged men: results of the Massachusetts Male Aging Study. J Clin Endocrinol Metab 73: 1016–1025

26. Henalla SM, Kirwan P, Castleden CM, Hutchins CJ, Breeson AJ (1988) The effect of pelvic floor exercises in the treatment of genuine urinary stress incontinence in women at two hospitals. Br J Obstet Gynaecol 95: 602–606

27. Hextall A (2000) Estrogens and lower urinary tract function. Maturitas 36: 83–9

28. Hextall A, Bidmead J, Cardozo L, Hooper R (2001) The impact of the menstrual cycle on urinary symptoms and the results of urodynamic investigation. Br J Obstet Gynaecol 108: 1193–1196

29. Jackson S, Shepherd A, Brookes S, Abrams P (1999) The effect of estrogen supplementation on post-menopausal urinary stress incontinence: a double-blind placebo-controlled trial. Br J Obstet Gynaecol 106: 711–718

30. Judge TG (1969) The use of quinestradiol in elderly incontinent women, a preliminary report. Gerontol Clin 11: 159–164

31. Keast JR, Saunders RJ (1998) Testosterone has potent, selective effects on the morphology of pelvic autonomic neurons which control the bladder, lower bowel and internal reproductive organs of the male rat. Neuroscience 85: 543–556

32. Kok AL, Burger CW, van de Weijer PH, Voetberg GA, Peters-Muller ER, Kenemans P (1999) Micturition complaints in postmenopausal women treated with continuously combined hormone replacement therapy: a prospective study. Maturitas 31: 143–149

33. Kuchel GA, Tannenbaum C, Greenspan SL, Resnick NM (2001) Can variability in the hormonal status of elderly women assist in the decision to administer oestrogens? J Womens Health Gend Based Med 10: 109–116

34. Kuroda H, Kohrogi T, Uchida N, Imai I, Terada N, Matsumoto K, Kitamura Y (1985) Urinary retention induced by estrogen injections in mice: an analytical model. J Urol 134: 1268–1270

35. Larsson B, Andersson KE, Batra S, Mattiasson A, Sjogren C (1984) Effects of estradiol on norepinephrine-induced contraction, alpha adrenoceptor number and norepinephrine content in the female rabbit urethra. J Pharmacol Exp Ther 229: 557–563

36. Milsom I, Abrams P, Cardozo L, Roberts RG, Thüroff J, Wein AJ (2001) How widespread are the symptoms of an overactive bladder and how are they managed? A population-based prevalence study. BJU Int 87: 760–766

37. Neaves WB, Johnson L, Porter JC, Parker CR Jr, Petty CS (1984) Leydig cell numbers, daily sperm production, and serum gonadotropin levels in aging men. J Clin Endocrinol Metab 59: 756–763

38. Nilsson K (1994) Urogenital estrogen deficiency in the postmenopuase (dissertation). Uppsala University: Uppsala, Sweden

39. Nilsson K, Heimer G (1992) Low-dose oestradiol in the treatment of urogenital oestrogen deficiency – a pharmacokinetic and pharmacodynamic study. Maturitas 15: 121–127

40. Notelovitz M (1995) Oestrogen therapy in the management of problems associated with urogenital aging: a simple diagnostic test and the effect of the route of hormone administration. Maturitas 22 [Suppl]: S31–S33

41. Ouslander JG, Greendale GA, Uman G, Lee C, Paul W, Schnelle J (2001) Effects of oral estrogen and progestin on the lower urinary tract among female nursing home residents. J Am Geriatr Soc 49: 803–807

42. Plas E, Berger P, Hermann M, Pflüger H (2000) Effects of aging on male fertility? Exp Gerontol 35: 543–551

43. Raz R, Stamm WE (1993) A controlled trial of intravaginal estriol in postmenopausal women with recurrent urinary tract infections. N Engl J Med 329: 753–756

44. Rizk DE, Raaschou T, Mason N, Berg B (2001) Evidence of progesterone receptors in the mucosa of the urinary bladder. Scand J Urol Nephrol 35: 305–309

45. Rolf C, Nieschlag E (2001) Reproductive functions, fertility and genetic risks of aging men. Exp Clin Endocrinol Diabetes 109: 68–74

46. Salmon UJ, Walter RI, Geist SH (1941) The use of estrogen in the treatment of dysuria and incontinence in post-menopausal women. Am J Obstet Gynecol 42: 845–851

47. Samsioe G (1998) Urogenital aging – a hidden problem. Am J Obstet Gynecol 178: S245–S249

48. Samsioe G, Jansson I, Mellstrom D, Svanborg A (1985) Occurrence, nature and treatment of urinary incontinence in a 70-year-old female population. Maturitas 7: 335–342

49. Sandford JP (1975) Urinarytract symptoms and infection. Ann Rev Med 26: 485–905
50. Shenfeld OZ, McCammon KA, Blackmore PF, Ratz PH (1999) Rapid effects of estrogen and progesterone on tone and spontaneous rhythmic contractions of the rabbit bladder. Urol Res 27: 386–392
51. Shenfield OZ, Blackmore PF, Morgan CW, Schlossberg SM, Jordan GH, Ratz PH (1998) Rapid effect of estradiol and progesterone on tone and spontaneuous rhythmic contractions of the rabbit bladder. Neurourol Urodynamics 17: 408–409
52. Shimonovitz S, Monga AK, Stanton SL (1997) Does the menstrual cycle influence cystometry? Int Urogynecol J Pelvic Floor Dysfunct 8: 213–215
53. Ulmsten U, Stormby N (1987) Evaluation of the urethral mucosa before and after oestrogen treatment in postmenopausal women with a new sampling technique. Gynecol Obstet Invest 24: 208–211
54. Vermeulen A, Kaufman JM (1995) Aging of the hypothalamo-pituitary-testicular axis in men. Horm Res 43: 25–28
55. Walter S, Kjaergaard B, Lose G, Andersen JT, Heisterberg L, Jakobson H (1990) Stress urinary incontinence in postmenopausal women treated with oral estrogen (estriol) and an α-adrenoceptor-stimulating agent (phenylpropanolamine): a randomized double-blind placebo-controlled study. Int Urogynecol J 1: 74–79
56. Walter S, Wolf H, Barlebo H, Jensen HK (1978) Urinary incontinence in postmenopausal women treated with estrogens: a double-blind clinical trial. Urol Int 33: 135–143
57. Wilson PD, Faragher B, Butler B, Bu'Lock D, Robinson EL, Brown AD (1987) Treatment with oral piperazine oestrone sulphate for genuine stress incontinence in postmenopausal women. Br J Obstet Gynaecol 94: 568–574
58. Yokoyama M, Fukutani K, Kawamura T, Shoji F, Ohtani M (1983) Stricture of the anterior urethra following estrogen therapy in patients with prostatic cancer. Urol Int 38: 247–250

Correspondence address: Eugen Plas, MD, Department of Urology and LBI for Urology & Andrology, Lainz Hospital, Wolkersbergenstrasse 1, A-1130 Vienna, Austria (E-mail: eugen.plas@wienkav.at).

Physiology and pathophysiology of bowel motility during aging and its therapeutic implications

J. Hammer

Department of Gastroenterology and Hepatology, University Clinic of Internal Medicine IV, General Hospital of Vienna, Vienna, Austria

Contents

1.   Intestinal motility

Intestinal motility comprises different aspects of movements of the intestine, namely movement of its wall and movement of its contents. Its coordinated action serves to optimise intestinal function by mixing of contents, delaying transit to secure digestion and absorption, acting as a storage site and evacuating stool. The mechanisms that control gastrointestinal (GI) motility are complex; the intrinsic nervous system (enteric nervous system) and prevertebral ganglia are key regulators, and central connections play a modulating role. Various circulating hormones also affect motility, and luminal contents regulate their own transport through the intestine as pointed out below.

Disorders of the neuromuscular apparatus of the GI tract are the commonest cause of GI symptoms and may manifest as constipation, diarrhoea, or fecal incontinence; bacterial overgrowth and diverticulosis also may be, at least in part, be related to disorders of GI motility. Signs and symptoms related to GI motor dysfunction are commonly reported to physicians by older patients. However, although biological changes have been described in elderly people, aging has relatively minor effects on GI motor functions, probably because of the large reserve capacity of the intestine (Camilleri et al. 2000, Firth et al. 2002). Other factors associated with aging, such as immobility and an impaired fluid balance, co-morbidity and medications, endocrine and metabolic disorders, might be of particular relevance in elderly people with intestinal motor dysfunction.

1.1 Physiology of small intestinal motility

In the fasting small bowel, a regular cycle of electrical activity alternating with phases of quiescence can be observed in the smooth muscle cells. This electrical activity also has its mechanical equivalent, phases of motor activity interrupted by phases of motor quiescence (Szurszewski 1969, Vantrappen et al. 1979). This fasting motility cycle consists of three phases: phase I, a period of quiescence when contractions are absent; phase II, during which sporadic contractions can be recorded; and phase III, the migrating motor complex (MMC), when the bowel contracts at its maximal frequency (Fig. 1). As the MMC moves distally down to the ileocolonic region, it sweeps the small intestine clear of the accumulated interdigestive debris and thus serves a so called 'house-keeper' function (Code and Schlegel 1999). Ingestion of a meal disrupts the interdigestive cycle, which is replaced by a postprandial pattern of sporadic, random contractions with apparently no regular pattern.

1.2 Physiology of large intestinal motility and anorectal function

In the large intestine, phases of contractile activity and phases of motor quiescence can be recorded apparently without a regular pattern (Bloom et al. 1968). A migrating motor complex such as in the small intestine does not exist in the colon. Other migrating motor patterns such as high amplitude propagated contractions (Narducci et al. 1987) – single, large amplitude contractions which migrate over long distances aborally – and a colonic motor complex, that has been described in dogs (Sarna et al. 1984), might be responsible for transport of luminal contents.

The normal fluid input into the human colon has been estimated as 1500–2000 ml per day (Phillips and Giller 1973) but the capacity of the colon to compensate for excess fluid is as high as 5–6 litres daily (Debongnie and Phillips 1978). Under physiological conditions the ascending colon and the transverse colon are major sites of storage and absorption (Hammer et al. 1990, Krevsky et al. 1986, Proano et al. 1990), whereas the descending colon and the rectosigmoid colon function mainly as conduits (Krevsky et al. 1986, Proano et al. 1990). Under pathological conditions, such as in Asiatic cholera (Camilleri et al. 2000) or carbohydrate malabsorption (Flourié et al. 1993), colonic fluid input can exceed 10 litres per day; when fluid input overwhelms storage capacity of the ascending and transverse colons (Hammer and Phillips 1993), both the descending colon as well as the

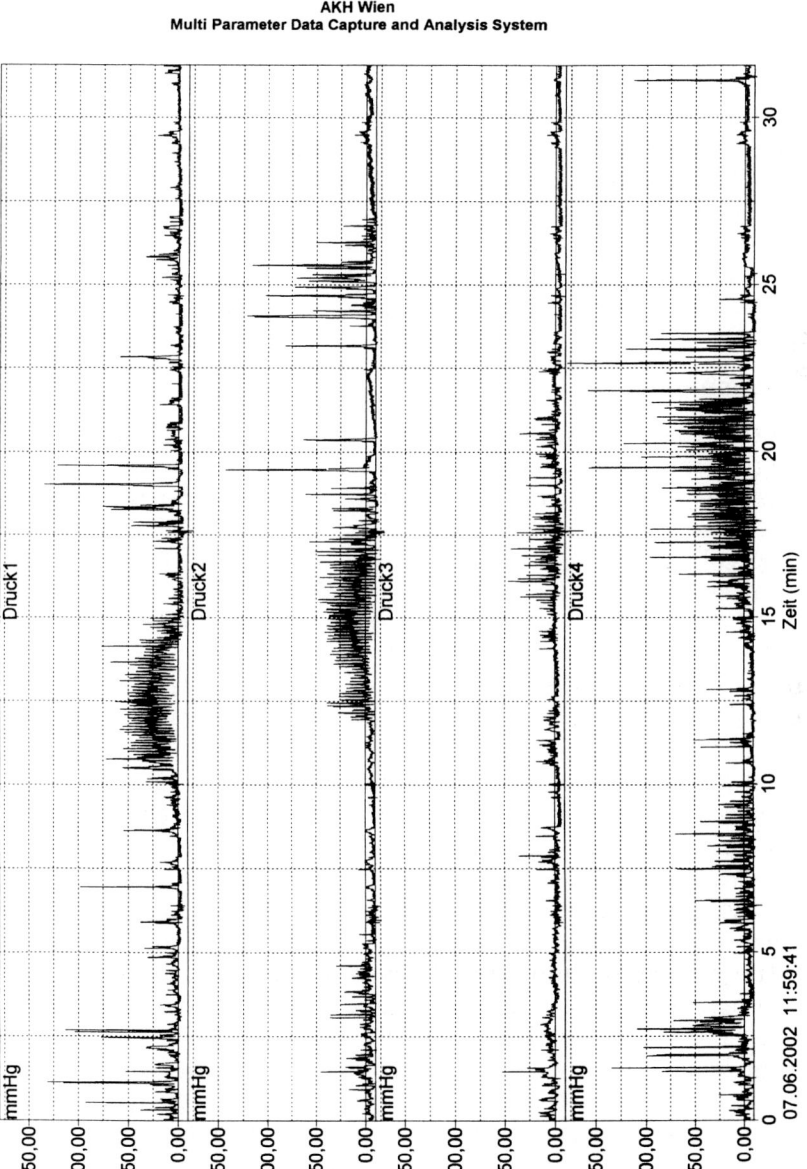

Fig. 1. Example of a normal fasting cycle in the small intestine of a 67 year old male. Four water perfused manometry ports are positioned (from top port to bottom) in the lower portion of the duodenum, 10 cm distally (at the ligament of Treitz), 20 cm and 25 cm distally of the proximal port. The migrating motor complex, MMC, migrates from proximal to distal and is characterised by regular contractions at maximal frequency. Phase II precedes the MMC, phase I (motor quiescence) follows after the MMC

rectosigmoid colon can provide reserve storage capacity that should allow additional mucosal absorption (Hammer et al. 1997).

The anorectum is concerned with storage and appropriate release of intestinal waste products. This involves the processes of detection and discrimination of rectal contents, retention, and controlled expulsion. The internal anal sphincter possesses a high level of tonic contraction that occludes the lumen and is responsible for most of the anal resting pressure. The external anal sphincter is a skeletal muscle that requires a conscious effort for contraction and its maximal contraction generates maximal squeeze pressure that can be measured during anorectal manometry. Defecation is a complex reflex mechanism that involves rectoanal musculature and perception, pelvic floor musculature, colonic musculature, and the muscles of the abdominal wall and thorax. Thus, the defecation reflex involves central nervous system pathways as well as local pathways in the enteric nerves. This coordinated function can be disturbed at many levels, and this may lead to either constipation or incontinence.

1.3   Regulation of intestinal motility

The mechanisms that regulate intestinal transport are complex, and our understanding of these mechanisms is yet far from complete. Extrinsic innervation as well as intrinsic innervation from the enteric nervous system influence intestinal motor function (Fig. 2), as do hormonal factors and the pacemaker cells, the so called interstitial cells of Cajal (Furness et al. 1999, Christensen 1992). Nutrients in the small intestinal lumen delay small intestinal transit compared with non-nutrient solutions (Read et al. 1980), and different nutrients such as fat and peptides have different effects on their own transport along the intestinal tract (Hammer et al. 1998a). Even small amounts of blood in the jejunal lumen, resembling minor upper GI bleeding, can accelerate transit through the proximal intestine compared with an isocaloric solution (Hammer et al. 1998b). Finally, the same nutrient can exert seemingly contrasting effects on GI transit when introduced into different sites in the intestine: fat that is delivered into the stomach or duodenum *delays* gastric emptying (Rao et al. 1996), whereas fat in the jejunum *accelerates* small intestinal transit (Hammer et al. 1998a). When fat is delivered into the ileum, however, gastric emptying and transit along the jejunum is *delayed*, a phenomenon that has been termed the "ileal break" mechanism (Spiller et al. 1984).

Neural control of GI motility is provided by an intrinsic nervous system, the enteric nervous system, that is able to mediate reflex activity in the absence of input from the central nervous system (Trendelenburg 1917, Kosterlitz and Lees 1964) and by constant modulation by prevertebral and central nervous input (Davison 1983) (Fig. 2). The bulk of the cell bodies of the enteric nervous system lie in the submucosa and in the intermuscular space between the circular and longitudinal muscle layers. Intestinal motor activity is also influenced by various regulatory peptides, which act via the

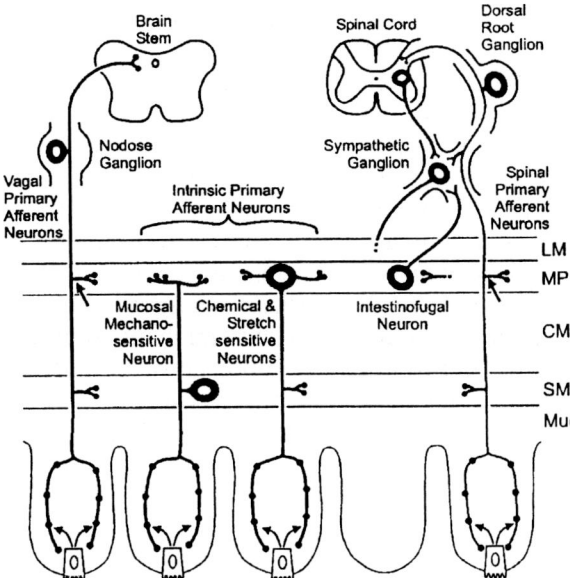

Fig. 2. Simplified diagram to illustrate the intrinsic nervous system and its extrinsic control (reprinted with permission from Furness JB, Kunze AA, Clerc N (1999) Nutrient tasting and signaling mechanisms in the gut II. The intestine as a sensory organ: neural, endocrine, and immune responses. Am J Physiol 277: G922–G928)

systemic circulation and are released from specialised cells located in the GI epithelia (Christensen 1998). Examples for such regulatory hormones are motilin and cholecystokinin. Motilin, a small peptide present in specialised cells in the stomach and upper small intestine as well as in the central nervous system, is released periodically in response to neural input and acts to initiate a migrating motility complex in the upper GI tract (Vantrappen et al. 1979) and accelerate GI transit (Bueno and Fioramonti 1994). Motilin also stimulates colonic motor complexes and giant motor complexes in the canine caecum (Sarna et al. 1988, Bickel and Belz 1988) and stimulates human colonic motor activity (Bueno and Fioramonti 1994). Another regulatory peptide, cholecystokinin (CKK), is present in endocrine cells of the upper small intestine, intestinal nerve fibres and the central nervous system and is released into the circulation in response to meals. Gastric emptying is delayed by CCK (Liddle et al. 1986) whereas a CCK-receptor antagonist, loxiglumide, accelerated both gastric emptying and colonic transit (Meyer et al. 1989).

2. Intestinal motility in elderly people

Overall, the intestine undergoes few physiologically and clinically significant changes with aging. Only minimal changes of small intestinal motility have been described in elderly subjects (Anuras and Sutherland 1984). As in young controls, the fasting motility cycle consists of three phases; the amplitude of contractions of phases II and III, the duration and the velocity of the MMC are unchanged (Anuras and Sutherland 1984). Only after a meal a decreased frequency of contractions has been observed (Anuras and Sutherland 1984); the physiologic consequences of this change are, however, relatively minor, as reflected by an unaltered small intestinal transit time with aging (Kupfer et al. 1985, Argenyi et al. 1995, Haboubi et al. 1988).

Large intestinal motility also undergoes relatively minor changes during aging. Motor activity in the sigmoid colon and rectum is not affected by age (Loening-Baucke and Anuras 1984). While Madsen reported an increase in colonic transit time with aging (Madsen 1992), others have found that in elderly persons intestinal transit time that is mainly determined by colonic residence time (Hammer and Phillips 1993) is comparable to healthy young adults (Melkersson et al. 1983, Brogna et al. 1999). However, brief physical inactivity prolongs colonic transit in elderly people (Liu et al. 1993).

Anorectal dysfunction has been reported in elderly subjects, mainly a decline of anal sphincter pressure at rest and at maximal squeeze (McHugh and Diamant 1987, Enck et al. 1989, Akervall et al. 1990). These age related changes might be responsible for the occurrence of fecal incontinence in elderly people. Some authors have also described a reduction in rectal sensation that impairs the sensation of rectal filling (Akervall et al. 1990), thus a decreased call for stool might abet the development of constipation or fecal incontinence.

3. Altered regulation of intestinal motility with aging

Earlier studies on aging in animal (Gabella 1989, Santer and Baker 1988) and human subjects (Gomes et al. 1997, Shankle et al. 1993) suggested that advanced age is associated with a significant decline in the number of neurons in the enteric nervous system. Recent studies, however, have used a staining method that quantified a more complete number of neurons in the myenteric plexus of the enteric nervous system (Johnson et al. 1998, Takahashi et al. 2000). These studies did not confirm a significant reduction of neurons in the old rat. However, aging has a pronounced effect on nitric oxide mediated inhibition of intestinal muscle: catalytic activity of nitric oxide synthase is reduced in the rat colon by advanced age (Takahashi et al. 2000). Moreover, the component of the relaxation of longitudinal muscle that is attributable to the effect of nitric oxide decreases with age both in the small and large intestine of the rat (Takeuchi et al. 1998). A decrease in this inhibitory mediator with age might explain a decrease in intrinsic inhibitory nerve input that has been shown in the colonic circular smooth muscle of elderly human subjects (Koch et al. 1991).

Besides these changes in intrinsic inhibition during aging, there is also a decline in the density of extrinsic fibres that project from the coeliac superior mesenteric ganglion to the enteric nervous system, (Baker et al. 1991). Finally, endocrine function may be altered with age, although data are sparse. The concentration of CCK in the guinea-pig duodenal mucosa increased with age, a fact that might reflect peripheral resistance to CCK (Poston et al. 1988); similarly, in 60–69 year old subjects the number of CCK-immunoreactive endocrine cells in the duodenum where significantly higher compared with 20–29 year old controls (Sandström and El-Salhy 1999).

4. Gastrointestinal symptoms in elderly people

Epidemiological studies have shown that the prevalence of gastrointestinal symptoms attributable to a dysfunction of gastrointestinal motility is high in elderly people. Talley et al. surveyed residents of Olmsted County in Minnesota, USA, aged 65–93 years, by means of a mailed questionnaire (Talley et al. 1992) (Fig. 3). 24% of the randomly selected elderly population reported chronic constipation, 14% had chronic diarrhoea, 24% frequent abdominal pain, and 7% had fecal incontinence (Talley et al. 1992). Similar prevalences were found in a 70-year old Danish population (Kay et al. 1993). The prevalence of fecal incontinence was 2% for solid stool leakage and 9% for liquid leakage in a population in western Sydney, Australia (Kalantar et al. 2002), and men and women were affected in approximately equal proportion. Prevalence of fecal incontinence increased with age in men from 8.4% among men in their fifties to 18.2% among men in their 80s (Roberts et al. 1999). Among the subjects with fecal incontinence, between 51% and 60% had concurrent urinary incontinence (Roberts et al. 1999). Finally, chronic gastrointestinal symptoms in elderly people interfered significantly with daily living and quality of life (O'Keefe et al. 1995).

4.1 Chronic constipation

The cause of constipation in elderly patients is often multifactorial and may include inactivity, inappropriate diet, depression and confusion, certain medications, and neuromuscular disorders (Wald 1993, Schiller 2001). Older subjects with constipation generally have prolonged recto-sigmoid transit (Evans et al. 1998) and pelvic floor dyssynergia and/or increased rectal compliance (Merkel et al. 1993). Table 1 summarises the therapeutic options in constipated patients. Since hypermagnesaemia may develop even in patients with normal renal function (Dharmarajan et al. 1999), the intake of magnesium salts should be avoided in elderly people.

Fecal impaction is a severe complication of constipation in elderly people and can cause fever, respiratory distress, or a decline in mental or

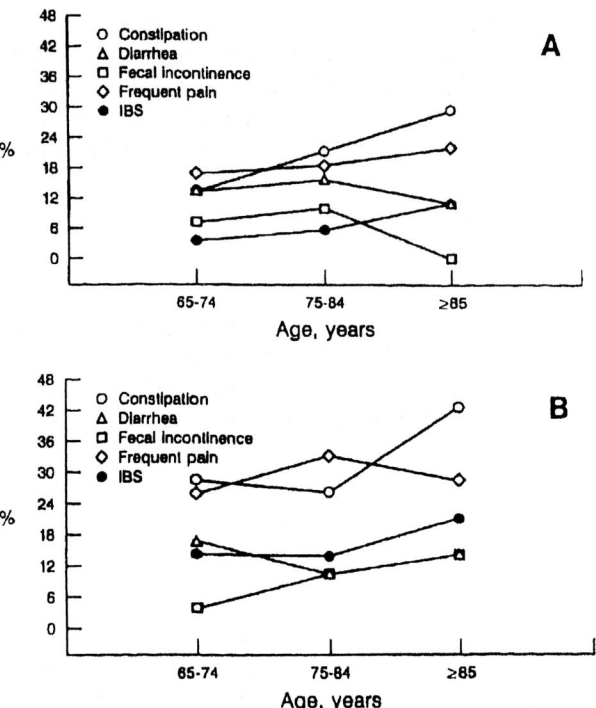

Fig. 3. Proportion of subjects with frequent abdominal pain, chronic constipation, chronic diarrhea, fecal incontinence, and symptoms of IBS (irritable bowel syndrome), by 10-year age group and gender (**A** men; **B** women). Reprinted with permission from Talley NJ, O'Keefe EA, Zinsmeister AR, Melton LJ 3rd (1992) Prevalence of gastrointestinal symptoms in the elderly: a population-based study. Gastroenterology 102: 895–901

Table 1. Therapeutic options in chronic constipated patients

First line:	Dietary and supplemental fiber
	Physical activity
	Bowel habit training and revision of concomitant therapy
Second line:	osmotic laxatives: e.g.: Sodium phosphate
	(Magnesium hydroxide)
	Lactulose syrup
	Polyethylene glycol (Macrogol)
	Stool softeners
Further:	Stimulant laxatives (for short term use): e.g.: Bisacodyl
	Senna
	Castor oil
	Suppositories: Glycerin
	Bisacodyl
	Enemas: Water
	Sodium phosphate

physical functioning. Its pathophysiology is complex, and reduced rectal perception, immobility and dementia are predisposing factors (Wrenn 1989). In populations at high risk, such as institutionalised or debilitated elderly people, mentally ill patients, patients with chronic renal failure or cancer, and neurologically impaired people, preventive measures should be undertaken (Wrenn 1989).

4.2   Chronic diarrhea

While in clinical practice diarrhea often is defined as a frequency greater than 3 bowel movements per day, elderly persons often use the term 'diarrhea' when they have rectal urgency (Talley et al. 1992). When an elderly patient presents with chronic diarrhea, specific potential causes (Table 2) and therapeutic considerations have to be kept in mind that might differ from other age groups: chronic diarrhea often occurs as side effect of a concomitant drug treatment (Ratnaike and Jones 1998) or as complication of concomitant disease such as diarrhea (Talley et al. 2001). Fecal impaction can manifest as so called 'overflow diarrhea', a condition that would exacerbate if treated with antidiarrhoeal agents.

Fluid loss during diarrhea can be considerable, and urinary concentration in elderly persons is less than in younger persons at the same degree of dehydration (Holt 2001). Mechanisms that lead to thirst might also be impaired with aging. Oral rehydration therapy and, in more severe cases, intravenous fluid therapy, should be started early.

4.3   Fecal incontinence

Symptoms of fecal incontinence are often present for years before patients seek medical attention. Patients are often reluctant to mention this symptom (Johanson and Lafferty 1996). They rather may report diarrhea or urgency, thus identifying fecal incontinence may require direct questions by the physician. Several conditions that are commoner in older patients can contribute to the development of fecal incontinence, such as altered rectal compliance, pelvic floor dysfunction, rectal sensory loss, and sphincter dysfunctions (Schiller

---

Table 2. Causes of chronic diarrhea in the elderly

- Drugs
- Fecal impaction
- Microscopic and collagenous colitis
- Inflammatory bowel disease
- Irritable bowel disease
- Cecliac sprue and other causes of malabsorption
- Others

2001). Neurological diseases and diabetic autonomic neuropathy also contribute to incontinence in elderly people.

Therapeutic options include both medical (for example, stimulating defecation at regular intervals, antidiarrhoeal drugs) and surgical options (for example, sphincteroplasty, pelvic floor repair). Psychological support is often needed and, of course, the underlying disease should be treated if possible.

4.4   Small intestinal bacterial overgrowth

Causes of small intestinal bacterial overgrowth may differ among patients, but in elderly patients a prolongation of small intestinal transit is a predisposing factor (Riordan et al. 1997). Although antibiotic therapy has been shown to be effective, treatment also should be directed towards correcting reversible causes of stasis (Firth and Prather 2002).

4.5   Diverticulosis

The pathogenesis of diverticular disease is yet not clear, although a relation between low dietary fibre and diverticular disease is well established (Farrel et al. 2001). A lack of fibre in the diet may lead to prolonged colonic transit and decreased stool volume, resulting in an increased intraluminal pressure. This pressure increase may press mucosa through defects in the colonic wall at sites of perforating arteries (Painter and Truelove 1964). The addition of indigestible fibres to the diet accelerates colonic transit, increases stool weight, and reduces intraluminal pressure in the sigmoid colon (Findlay et al. 1974).

5.   Closing remarks

Dysfunction of the small and large intestinal motility and regulation of neuromuscular function have been observed during aging. However, physiological and clinical significant changes during aging are minimal, probably because of the large reserve capacity of the small and large intestine. However, gastrointestinal problems that can be attributed to gastrointestinal motility disorders are often reported by elderly persons. This is probably due to other factors that are more prevalent during aging, such as immobility, concomitant use of medication, and disease. Specific aspects have to be taken into account in the diagnosis and treatment of gastrointestinal motor disorders in elderly patients.

6.   References

1. Akervall S, Nordgren S, Fasth S, Oresland T, Pettersson K, Hulten L (1990) The effects of age, gender, and parity on rectoanal functions in adults. Scand J Gastroenterol 25: 1247–1256
2. Anuras S, Sutherland J (1984) Small intestinal manometry in healthy elderly subjects. J Am Geriatr Soc 32: 581–583

3. Argenyi EE, Soffer EE, Madsen MT, Berbaum KS, Walkner WO (1995) Scintigraphic evaluation of small bowel transit in healthy subjects: inter and intrasubject variability. Am J Gastroenterol 90: 938–942

4. Baker DM, Watson SP, Santer RM (1991) Evidence for a decrease in sympathetic control of intestinal function in the aged rat. Neurobiol Aging 12: 363–365

5. Banwell JG, Pierce NF, Mitra RC, Brigham KL, Caranasos GH, Keimowitz RI (1970) Intestinal fluid and electrolyte transport in human cholera. J Clin Invest 49: 183–185

6. Bickel M, Belz U (1988) Motilin and a synthetic enkephalin induce colonic motor complexes (CMC) in the conscious dog. Peptides 9: 501–507

7. Bloom AA, Lopresti P, Farrar JT (1968) Motility of the intact human colon. Gastroenterology 54: 232–240

8. Brogna A, Ferrara R, Bucceri AM, Lanteri E, Catalano F (1999) Influence of aging on gastrointestinal transit time. An ultrasonographic and radiologic study. Invest Radiol 34: 357–359

9. Bueno L, Fioramonti J (1994) Neurohormonal control of intestinal transit. Reprod Nutr Dev 34: 513–525

10. Camilleri M, Lee JS, Viramontes B, Bharucha AE, Tangalos EG (2000) Insights into the pathophysiology and mechanisms of constipation, irritable bowel syndrome, and diverticulosis in older people. J Am Geriatr Soc 48: 1142–1150

11. Christensen J (1992) Commentary on the morphological identification of the interstitial cells of Cajal. J Auton Nerv Syst 37: 75–88

12. Christensen J (1998) Intestinal motor physiology. In: Feldmann M, Scharschmidt BF, Sleisenger MH, Klein S (eds) Sleisinger & Fordtran's gastrointestinal and liver disease: pathophysiology/diagnosis/management. W. B. Saunders Company 6th edn, vol 2, pp 1437–1450

13. Code CF, Schlegel JF (2001) The gastrointestinal interdigestive houskeeper: motor correlates of the interdigestive myoelectric complex of the dog. In: Daniel EE (ed) Proc. Fourth International Symposium on GI Motility. Mitchell Press: Vancouver

14. Davison JS (1998) Innervation of the gastrointestinal tract. In: Christensen J, Wingate DL (eds) A guide to gastrointestinal motility. Chapter 1, Wright PSG: Bristol, London, Boston, pp 147

15. Debongnie JC, Phillips SF (1978) Capacity of the human colon to absorb fluid. Gastroenterology 74: 698–703

16. Dharmarajan TS, Patel B, Varshneya N (1999) Cathartic-induced life threatening hypermagnesemia in a 90-year-old woman with apparent normal renal function. J Am Geriatr Soc 47: 1039–1040

17. Enck P, Kuhlbusch R, Lubke H, Frieling T, Erckenbrecht JF (1989) Age and sex and anorectal manometry in incontinence. Dis Colon Rectum 32: 1026–1030

18. Evans JM, Fleming KC, Talley NJ, Schleck CD, Zinsmeister AR, Melton LJ 3rd (1998) Relation of colonic transit to functional bowel disease in older people: a population-based study. J Am Geriatr Soc 46: 83–87

19. Farrel RJ, Farrell JJ, Morrin MM (2001) Diverticular disease in the elderly. Gastroenterol Clin North Am 30: 475–496

20. Findlay JM, Smith AN, Mitchell WD, Anderson AJ, Eastwood MA (1974) Effects of unpreocessed bran on colon function in normal subjects and in diverticular disease. Lancet 1: 146–149

21. Firth M, Prather CM (2002) Gastrointestinal motility problems in the elderly patient. Gastroenterology 122: 1688–1700

22. Flourié B, Briet F, Florent Ch, Pellier P, Maurel M, Rambaud JC (1993) Can diarrhoea induced by lactulose be reduced by prolonged ingestion of lactulose? Am J Clin Nutr 58: 369–375

23. Furness JB, Kunze AA, Clerc N (1999) Nutrient tasting and signaling mechanisms in the gut II. The intestine as a sensory organ: neural, endocrine, and immune responses. Am J Physiol 277: G922–G928

24. Gabella G (1989) Fall in the number of myenteric neurons in aging guinea pigs. Gastroenterology 96: 1487–1493

25. Gomes OA, de Souza RR, Liberti EA (1997) A preliminary investigation of the effects of aging on the nerve cell number in the myenteric ganglia of the human colon. Gerontology 43: 210–217

26. Haboubi NY, Hudson P, Rahman Q, Lee GS, Ross A (1988) Small intestinal transit time in the elderly. Lancet 1: 933

27. Hammer HF, Fine KD, SantaAna CA, Porter JL, Schiller LR, Fordtran JS (1990) Carbohydrate malabsorption. Its measurement and its contribution to diarrhoea. J Clin Invest 86: 1936–1944

28. Hammer J, Hammer K, Kletter K (1998a) Lipids infused into the jejunum accelerate small intestinal transit but delay ileocolonic transit of solids and liquids. Gut 43: 111–116

29. Hammer J, Lang K, Kletter K (1998b) Accelerated right colonic emptying after simulated upper gut haemorrhage. Am J Gastroent 93: 628–631

30. Hammer J, Phillips SF (1993) Fluid loading of the human colon: effects on segmental transit and stool composition. Gastroenterology 105: 988–998

31. Hammer J, Pruckmayer M, Bergmann H, Kletter K, Gangl A (1997) The distal colon provides reserve storage capacity during colonic fluid overload. Gut 41: 658–663

32. Holt PR (2001) Diarrhea and malabsorption in the elderly. Gastroenterol Clin North Am 30: 427–444

33. Johanson JF, Lafferty J (1996) Epidemiology of fecal incontinence: the silent affliction. Am J Gastroenterol 91: 33–36

34. Johnson RJ, Schemann M, Santer RM, Cowen T (1998) The effects of age on the overall population and on subpopulations of myenteric neurons in the rat small intestine. J Anat 192: 479–488

35. Kalantar JS Howell S, Talley NJ (2002) Prevalence of faecal incontinence and associated risk factors; an underdiagnosed problem in the Australian community? Med J Aust 176: 54–57

36. Kay L, Jorgensen T, Schultz-Larsen K (1993) Colon related symptoms in a 70-year-old Danish population. J Clin Epidemiol 46: 1445–1449

37. Koch TR, Carney A, Go VLW, Szurszewski JH (1991) Inhibitory neuropeptides and intrinsic inhibitory innervation of descending human colon. Dig Dis Sci 36: 712–718

38. Kosterlitz HW, Lees GM (1964) Pharmacological analysis of intrinsic intestinal reflexes. Pharmacol Rev 16: 301–339

39. Krevsky B, Malmud LS, D'Ercole F, Maurer AH, Fisher RS (1986) Colonic transit scintigraphy. A physiologic approach to the quantitative measurement of colonic transit in humans. Gastroenterology 91: 1102–1112

40. Kupfer RM, Heppell M, Haggith JW, Bateman DN (1985) Gastric emptying and smallbowel transit rate in the elderly. J Am Geriatr Soc 33: 340–343

41. Liddle RA, Morita ET, Conrad CK, Williams JA (1986) Regulation of gastric emptying in humans by cholecystokinin. J Clin Invest 77: 992–996

42. Liu F, Kondo T, Toda Y (1993) Brief physical inactivity prolongs colonic transit time in elderly active men. Int J Sports Med 14: 465–746
43. LoeningBaucke V, Anuras S (1984) Sigmoidal and rectal motility in healthy elderly. J Am Geriatr Soc 32: 887–891
44. Madsen JL (1992) Effects of gender, age, and body mass index on gastrointestinal transit times. Dig Dis Sci 37: 1548–1553
45. McHugh SM, Diamant NE (1987) Effect of age, gender, and parity on anal canal pressures. Contribution of impaired anal sphincter function to fecal incontinence. Dig Dis Sci 32: 726–736
46. Melkersson M, Andersson H, Bosaeus I, Falkheden T (1983) Intestinal transit time in constipated and nonconstipated geriatric patients. Scand J Gastroenterol 18: 593–597
47. Merkel IS, Locher J, Burgio K, Towers A, Wald A (1993) Physiologic and psychologic characteristics of an elderly population with chronic constipation. Am J Gastroenterol 88: 1854–1859
48. Meyer BM, Werth BA, Beglinger C, Hildebrand P, Jansen JBMJ, Zach D, Rovati LC, Stalder GA (1989) Role of cholecystokinin regulation of gastrointestinal motor function. Lancet 2: 12–15
49. Narducci F, Bassotti G, Gaburri M, Morelli A (1987) Twentyfour hour manometric recording of colonic motor activity in healthy man. Gut 28: 17–25
50. O'Keefe EA, Talley NJ, Zinsmeister AR, Jacobsen SJ (1995) Bowel disorders impair functional status and quality of life in the elderly: a population-based study. J Gerontol A Biol Sci Med Sci 50: M184–M189
51. Painter NS, Truelove SC (1964) The intraluminal pressure patterns in diverticulosis of the colon. Part I. Resting patterns of pressure. Part II. The effect of morphine. Part III. The effect of prostigmin. Part IV. The effect of pethidine and probanthine. Gut 5: 201
52. Phillips SF, Giller J (1973) The contribution of the colon to electrolyte and water conservation in man. J Lab Clin Med 81: 733–746
53. Poston GJ, Singh P, Draviam EJ, Upp JR Jr, Thompson JC (1988) Development and age-related changes in pancreatic cholecystokinin receptors and duodenal cholecystokinin in guinea pigs. Mech Aging Dev 46: 59–66
54. Proano M, Camilleri M, Phillips SF, Prown ML, Thomforde GM (1990) Transit of solids through the human colon: regional quantification in the unprepared bowel. Am J Physiolo 258: G856–862
55. Rao SS, Lu C, Schulze-Delrieu K (1996) Duodenum as a immediate brake to gastric outflow: a videofluoroscopic and manometric assessment. Gastroenterology 110: 740–747
56. Ratnaike RN, Jones TE (1998) Mechanisms of drug-induced diarrhea in the elderly. Drugs Aging 13: 245–253
57. Read NW, Miles CA, Fisher D, Holgate AM, Kime ND, Mitchell MA, Reeve AM, Roche TB, Walker M (1980) Transit of a meal through the stomach, small intestine and colon in normal subjects and its role in the pathogenesis of diarrhea. Gastroenterology 79: 1276–1282
58. Riordan SM, McIver CJ, Wakefield D, Bolin TD, Duncombe VM, Thomas MC (1997) Small intestinal bacterial overgrowth in the symptomatic elderly. Am J Gastroenterol 92: 47–51
59. Roberts RO, Jacobsen SJ, Reilly WT, Pemberton JH, Lieber MM, Talley NJ (1999) Prevalence of combined fecal and urinary incontinence: a community-based study. J Am Geriatr Soc 47: 837–841

60. Sandström O, El-Salhy M (1999) Aging and endocrine cells of human duodenum. Mech Aging Devel 108: 39–48
61. Santer RM, Baker DM (1988) Enteric neuron numbers and sizes in Auerbach's plexus in the small and large intestine of adult and aged rats. J Auton Nerv Syst 25: 59–67
62. Sarna SK, Condon R, Cowles V (1984) Colonic migrating and nonmigrating motor complexes in dogs. Am J Physiol 246: G355–G360
63. Sarna S, Condon RE, Cowles V (1988) Giant migrating contractions in the canine caecum. Am J Physiol 254: G595–G601
64. Schiller LR (2001) Constipation and fecal incontinence in the elderly. Gastroenterol Clin North Am 30: 497–515
65. Shankle WR, Landing BH, Ang SM, Chui H, Villarreal-Engelhardt G, Zarow C (1993) Studies of the enteric nervous system in Alzheimer disease and other dementias of the elderly: enteric neurons in Alzheimer disease. Mod Pathol 6: 10–14
66. Spiller RC, Trotman IF, Higgins BE, Ghatei MA, Grimble GK, Lee YC, Bloom SR (1984) The ileal brakeinhibition of jejunal motility after ileal fat perfusion in man. Gut 25: 365–374
67. Szurszewski JH (1969) A migrating electric complex of the canine small intestine. Am J Physiol 217: 1757–1763
68. Takeuchi T, Niioka S, Yamaji M, Okishio Y, Ishii T, Nishio H, Takatsuji K, Hata F (1998) Decrease in participation of nitric oxide in nonadrenergic, noncholinergic relaxation of rat intestine with age. Jpn J Pharmacol 78: 293–302
69. Takahashi T, Qoubaitary A, Owyang C, Wiley JW (2000) Decreased expression of nitric oxide syndthase in the colonic myenteric plexus of aged rats. Brain Res 883: 15–21
70. Talley NJ, O'Keefe EA, Zinsmeister AR, Melton LJ 3rd (1992) Prevalence of gastrointestinal symptoms in the elderly: a population-based study. Gastroenterology 102: 895–901
71. Talley NJ, Young LJ, Bytzer P, Hammer J, Leemon M, Jones M, Horowitz M (2001) Impact of chronic gastrointestinal symptoms in diabetes mellitus on health-related quality of life. Am J Gastroenterol 96: 71–76
72. Trendelenburg P (1917) Physiologische und pharmakologische Versuche über die Dünndarmperistaltik. Naunyn Schmiedebergs Arch Exp Pathol Pharmakol 81: 55–129
73. Vantrappen G, Janssens J, Peeters TL, Bloom SR, Christofides ND, Hellemans J (1979) Motility and the interdigestive migrating motor complex in man. Dig Dis Sci 24: 497–500
74. Wald A (1993) Constipation in elderly patients. Pathogenesis and management. Drugs Aging 3: 220–231
75. Wrenn K (1989) Fecal impaction. N Engl J Med 321: 658–662

Correspondence address: Johann Hammer, MD, Department of Gastroenterology and Hepatology, University Clinic of Internal Medicine IV, General Hospital of Vienna, Währinger Gürtel 18-20, A-1090 Vienna, Austria (E-mail: Johann.Hammer@univie.ac.at).

Index

SpringerMedicine

Mohammad R. Nowrousian (ed.)

Recombinant Human Erythropoietin (rhEPO) in Clinical Oncology

Scientific and Clinical Aspects of Anemia in Cancer

2002. IX, 502 pages. 66 figures, partly in colour.
Hardcover **EUR 98,–**
(Recommended retail price) Net-price subject to local VAT.
ISBN 3-211-83661-6

Anemia is a frequent complication of cancer and its treatment. A number of clinical studies shows that the impact of anemia is much greater than previously thought. Beyond clinical symptoms, anemia significantly impairs physical and metabolic functions as well as patients' activity, well-being and quality of life. Life expectancy is also affected.

In this book, written by a group of outstanding international experts, the current knowledge on anemia in cancer and its treatment with rhEPO is presented and future developments are discussed. Based on a broad spectrum of topics, the book describes the scientific and clinical aspects of anemia in various fields of oncology and gives diagnostic and therapeutic recommendations on when and how to use rhEPO.

The book will serve as an authentic and essential source of information for radiotherapists, oncologists, hematologists, internists, pediatricians, surgeons, specialists in transfusion or laboratory medicine and pharmacologists.

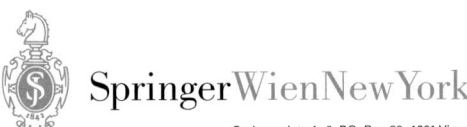

SpringerWienNewYork

Sachsenplatz 4–6, P.O. Box 89, 1201 Vienna, Austria, Fax +43.1.330 24 26, e-mail: books@springer.at, Internet: **www.springer.at**
Haberstraße 7, 69126 Heidelberg, Germany, Fax +49.6221.345-4229, e-mail: orders@springer.de
P.O. Box 2485, Secaucus, NJ 07096-2485, USA, Fax +1.201.348-4505, e-mail: orders@springer-ny.com
Eastern Book Service, 3–13, Hongo 3-chome, Bunkyo-ku, Tokyo 113-8480, Japan, Fax +81.3.38 18 08 64, e-mail: orders@svt-ebs.co.jp

SpringerMedicine

Ines Mader, Patrizia R. Fürst-Weger,
Robert M. Mader, Elisabeth I. Semenitz,
Robert Terkola, Sabine M. Wassertheurer

Extravasation of Cytotoxic Agents

Compendium for Prevention and Management

Translated from German by Birte Twisselmann.
2003. IX, 253 pages. 1 figure. With cd-rom and 5 work sheets
Hardcover **EUR 49,–**
(Recommended retail price) Net-price subject to local VAT.
ISBN 3-211-83859-7

Extravasation of cytotoxic drugs can lead to serious complications
during tumour therapy. This volume is intended as an aid to assess
the situation quickly and conclusively should this emergency
occur. The substance specific section of the book provides detailed
instructions for how to deal with 49 cytotoxic agents so that targeted measures can be started at once. The general section provides
comprehensive information on prevention, general measures to be
taken in case of extravasation, specific antidotes, and documen-
tation. For support during everyday clinical practice, the book is
accompanied by a template for an extravasation kit, tables, docu-
mentation sheets, and patient information.

The book is the outcome of a consensus of an interdisciplinary
working group that has collected and systematically reviewed all
published literature on the topic. The practical instructions are accompanied by a review of the literature to enable readers to study
source materials via the original published studies.

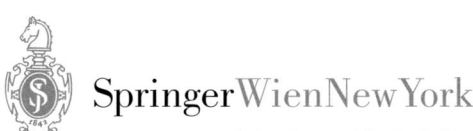

SpringerWienNewYork

Sachsenplatz 4–6, P.O. Box 89, 1201 Vienna, Austria, Fax +43.1.330 24 26, e-mail: books@springer.at, Internet: **www.springer.at**
Haberstraße 7, 69126 Heidelberg, Germany, Fax +49.6221.345-4229, e-mail: orders@springer.de
P.O. Box 2485, Secaucus, NJ 07096-2485, USA, Fax +1.201.348-4505, e-mail: orders@springer-ny.com
Eastern Book Service, 3–13, Hongo 3-chome, Bunkyo-ku, Tokyo 113-8480, Japan, Fax +81.3.38 18 08 64, e-mail: orders@svt-ebs.co.jp